HUNGRY FOR HEALTH

**157 delicious, nutritious dishes
to help
prevent and reverse disease**

Susan Silberstein, PhD

Copyright © 2005 by Susan Silberstein

ISBN 0-7414-2368-5

Published by:

INFINITY
PUBLISHING.COM

1094 New DeHaven Street, Suite 100
West Conshohocken, PA 19428-2713
Info@buybooksontheweb.com
www.buybooksontheweb.com
Toll-free (877) BUY BOOK
Local Phone (610) 941-9999
Fax (610) 941-9959

Printed in the United States of America

Printed on Recycled Paper

Published February 2005

"A brilliant accomplishment...presenting real world, tried and true recipes for those people who are serious about promotion of health and prevention of disease."
—Richard DuBois, MD, FACP
Past President, Medical Association of Atlanta

"Your complete source for recipes that distill all the dietary elements shown by research as being essential for optimal health and disease prevention. Keep it handy and become healthier!"
—M. Warren Peary
Author, *The Ten Biggest Diet Myths and Greatest Health Secrets Revealed*

"A practical, well-constructed collection of informative data, valuable dietary guidelines, and life-changing recipes."
—Richard M. Goldfarb, MD, FACS
Medical Director, Bucks County Clinical Research, Inc.

"... a necessity for anyone interested in healthy eating -- from the beginner to the committed vegetarian -- ....healthy cooking as it should be -- fun, easy, delicious and exciting! Every food lover should own this book!"
—Pamela A. Popper, PhD, ND
Executive Director, The Wellness Forum

To Tony

TABLE OF CONTENTS

PREFACE

I have two confessions to make: First, I am not a chef. Second, my recipes are not so original. *So why am I writing a cookbook?*

Actually, it's the last thing I ever thought I'd write. But here's how it came about: Over the last quarter century, I and my staff at the Center for Advancement in Cancer Education have provided dietary guidance to more than 25,000 clients — for cancer prevention, for prevention of recurrence and for support during or after treatment. We teach what to avoid, what to eat, why to eat it, how to prepare it. To help people learn, we have often recommended healthful recipe books.

However, our tools have been inadequate. Several of our favorite books are out of print. Some books list ingredients but no quantities. Some list quantities but no yield. Some use ingredients that are hard to find. Some give recipes that are very difficult to prepare. Some supposedly healthful recipe books include ingredients or cooking methods we consider inappropriate for those seeking health. The really healthful ones include recipes that are tough on the taste buds. Some books feature only uncooked recipes — too weird. Others feature all cooked ones — too hard on the digestion. Most health food recipe books are all vegetarian. The real world occasionally eats animal protein. Recipes that would do for the entire family – and (dare I say it?) mealtime guests — were scarce indeed. Our clients who wanted to comply were getting really bored with juices and salads. We found ourselves dictating recipes day after day. Everyone was somewhat frustrated.

So here it is: A *mesclun* of recipes from a variety of sources to address a variety of needs. Something for everyone. Some recipes are uncooked; some are cooked. Some are straight from "scratch"; some use shortcuts. Most are vegetarian; some have animal protein in them. A few contain flour or dairy; most do not. Not only are these recipes *not bad* for you — nearly all are *really good* for you. The recipes are borrowed, adapted, and rarely, if at all, the way they appeared at the source. But they are all tested — both by those passionate about health and by those passionate about food.

Most of these recipes are really easy to make. I am finally out to debunk the myth that states "If it's good for you it's got to be annoying to prepare!" I figure if people are going to eat what I want them to eat, then *what I want them to eat better be easy to make and easy to like.* As Andrew Weil, MD, pointed out, "Food that is healthy and food that gives pleasure are not mutually exclusive." So the three guiding principles for the recipes in this book are these: HEALTHFUL, SIMPLE, and TASTY. I will add that EVERY INGREDIENT SHOULD BE AS FRESH, PURE AND ORGANIC AS POSSIBLE — whether or not that is stated explicitly in the recipe. (For example, if a recipe requires water, I write "water." My readers should assume that I mean the purest spring or distilled or filtered water possible to obtain. If a recipe states "apples," know that I mean organic apples.) Let me also mention that you should feel free to add any spices you like — they have medicinal value.

I have another principle that I tell my clients: YOU HAVE TO CHEAT ON MY DIET. Yes, it's absolutely required! Because if life isn't worth living, why bother fighting to be well? So there's Christmas and Easter and your birthday and that special invitation. It's fine to cheat occasionally. The question is, what do you do for 19 out of the 21 meals per week? Hopefully, a lot of what you'll do lies nestled in the pages of *Hungry for Health*.

I wish to express my special thanks to the following:

Natalie Dyen for her incredible help and competent training in format and graphics

Anne Stokes Hochberg for her generous assistance with layout

Lucie Urban for her kind and patient technical support

All those who shared their recipes or helped test mine, including **Dr. Risa Broudy, Sherry Milner, Christina Pirello, Judy Levin, Paula Krasnoff, Joel Odhner**, **Ruth Harp**, and **Ethan Jarvis**

My Golden Retriever, **Butterscotch** — who has always eaten better than most humans – who was steadfastly willing to taste, day and night, any and all recipes, and who gave me his wholehearted approval on *every single one*

The researchers, clinicians, and recovered

patients whose books served as my sources (see references) and from whom I adapted or borrowed recipes

And finally, the thousands of health consumers I have been privileged to encounter who begged me to complete this project.

It is my pleasure to donate profits from sales of this book to help support the wonderful work of the Center for Advancement in Cancer Education, a national not-for-profit organization that specializes in dietary and lifestyle training for cancer prevention, prevention of recurrence, and support during treatment.

Center for Advancement in Cancer Education
300 E. Lancaster Ave. #100
Wynnewood, PA 19096
610-642-4810 (phone)
610-896-6339 (fax)
BeatCancer.org
info@beatcancer.org

INTRODUCTION: THE BASICS

THE BASICS

Many of my patients have said to me, "I don't understand how I got sick; I've always eaten healthy." My answer to them is always two-fold: First, it may not be so much what you're eating as what's eating you. (After all, "stressed" spelled backwards is "desserts.") Second, there are probably as many definitions of "good nutrition" as there are people trying to define it.

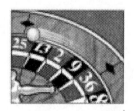 For years, Americans have been playing Dietary Roulette. We have all heard about the Atkins Diet, the Zone Diet, the Mediterranean Diet, the South Beach Diet, the Hollywood Diet, the Eat-Right-for-Your-Blood-Type Diet, the Eat-Right-for-Your-Astrological-Sign Diet, the High-Carb-Low-Fat-Diet, the High-Protein-Low-Carb-Diet.... We've certainly been hearing a lot of conflicting information about all these diet and nutrition fads. But let's get down to the science.

So many diets, so little health

More and more, nutritional science investigations have been pointing to a significant connection between our diets and our health. One thing is becoming abundantly clear: Americans aren't very healthy. 23 million Americans have already been diagnosed with cancer. Each year, a million more are diagnosed, and within five years 500,000 will have died of it. The lifetime risk for cancer is now one in two Americans and two in three American families.

More grim statistics: 41 million Americans have heart disease. Over one million have a heart attack every year, and half a million heart attack victims die each year. 18 million Americans have been diagnosed with diabetes, and within two generations that number is expected to double. Sixty-four percent of Americans are overweight or obese; obesity correlates with all three of the killer diseases I just mentioned. According to the World Health Federation, over 70 percent of all deaths in the United States are diet related.

Are you digging your grave with your fork?

Yes, the evidence demonstrates that Americans are digging themselves into early graves with their forks — in fact, very early! Our children are increasingly unhealthy, too. One out of two children born today will develop heart disease. One out of 2.5 will be diagnosed with cancer. 20 million children are obese. By the age of 12, 70 percent of all American children will have developed the beginning stages of hardening of the arteries. And at the current rates, of those children born in the year 2000, a full 50 percent will have type 2 adult onset diabetes by the time they reach 30!

Overfed and undernourished

What is the reason for this sorry state of affairs? In large measure, their diets! It doesn't take an arms inspector to spot one of the biggest weapons of mass destruction facing Americans today: It's the school lunch — full of saturated fat, cholesterol and sugar, and devoid of any real nutrition. The acronym for the Standard American Diet is very SAD indeed. We are, SADly, overfed but undernourished. In fact, a recent three-day study conducted by the U.S. Department of Agriculture (USDA) showed that out of 21,500 persons, *not a single one* consumed the RDA for 10 essential nutrients! And, of course, the "recommended daily amount" is pitifully low, at levels just enough to prevent deficiency diseases like scurvy, rickets and beriberi. Basically, the RDA is the nutritional equivalent of the minimum wage.

Pyramids and portion control

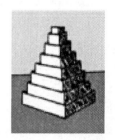

Our government has been trying to help. In 1992, the USDA issued a food guide pyramid in an effort to wean Americans off fat. Unfortunately, that pyramid conveyed a sense that all carbohydrates are harmless. It did not distinguish between refined carbohydrates and complex carbs from whole foods. Nor did it distinguish between saturated animal fats and unsaturated plant-based fats. Or between high-fat and lean sources of protein.

Now, a decade later, we have been offered a far superior healthy eating pyramid from Dr. Walter Willett of the Harvard School of Public Health. The new pyramid promotes mostly whole grains, plant oils, fresh fruits and vegetables, raw nuts, and legumes. It includes fish, poultry, eggs and dairy, but recommends very limited use of saturated fats like red meat and butter, and greatly restricts refined carbohydrates like bread, pasta and sugar. It also emphasizes another problem of the American diet: **portion distortion**! Americans simply eat two to four times what is recommended. Now, the Harvard pyramid is not just another fad diet, and not just another weight-loss gimmick. It is basic to lifetime human health.

Four principles of healthy eating

There's only one problem. Pyramids don't prevent disease; healthy habits do. So let's look at the four most fundamental principles of healthy eating and see how simply they can be integrated into our lifestyles.

1: Eat primitive

First and foremost — and despite the *latest* information — the best advice is still the *oldest*: EAT PRIMITIVE.

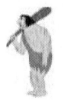 That's what Drs. Boyd Eaton and Melvin Konner suggested in an article, published in the *New England Journal of Medicine* in January of 1985, called "Paleolithic Nutrition." According to anthropologists, humanity has been around as a genus for about two million years and as a species for about 40,000 years. All that time we ate a consistent way — the hunter-gatherer society diet — until about 150 or 200 years ago, when the Industrial Revolution came along, and modern food processing techniques began refining the Western diet and stripping it

of most of its nutrients. But one to two centuries are a mere drop in the proverbial evolutionary bucket — hardly enough time for our genes to adapt to this dramatic departure from long-established dietary patterns. The result: chronic killer diseases like heart disease, cancer, and diabetes — conditions that are virtually unknown in traditional cultures that still eat a primitive diet today.

And what is that diet? A lot of plants:

* Roots and fruits
* Greens and beans
* Seeds and weeds

Plus some fish or wild game.

Our modern diet is quite different:

* Meats and sweets
* Pies and fries
* Chips and dips
* Cakes and shakes

Put a primitive in a supermarket, and, with the exception of the fish and produce department, she's not likely to find anything she can recognize as food; our cells are in a similar predicament.

The skinny on fats

One key difference between the modern and paleolithic diets is the fat content, especially saturated animal fats — which definitely contribute to chronic degenerative disease. As I often quip, double cheeseburger, triple bypass. Or, said another way, the Golden Arches are one step away from the Pearly Gates. A recent film, "Super Size Me," documents the near disastrous health consequences experienced by a man who eats in McDonald's for 30 days in a row.

Fats are important in three ways -- in terms of amount, type and quality. The diet of our ancestors was much lower in fat, compared with the 40%-60% we consume today. And in the primitive diet, only about 35% of the fat consumed was the dangerous saturated kind, as opposed to the 99% saturated fats in the animal foods we consume today.

Unsaturated fats are often combinations of omega 3, 6 or 9 fatty acids. Although all have value, high omega 6 fats tend to down-regulate the immune system, high omega 3s enhance immune function, and omega 9s are neutral. In hunter-gatherer diets, the ratio of omega 6 fatty acids to omega 3s was about 1 to 1 or at most 2 to 1 — a nice balance for the immune system. However, the ratios in our western diet today are at least 20 to 1, and some researchers say 30 to 1, in favor of omega 6 and against your immune system.

	Omega 6	Omega3
Primitive	1	1
Modern	20	1

Ratio of Omega 6 to Omega 3 Dietary Fats

Expressed oils like corn oil, cottonseed oil, soybean oil, sunflower oil, and safflower oil are high in omega 6s and should be avoided. Good sources of omega 3s are fish, ground flaxseeds, wild game, free range poultry and their eggs, sea vegetables, raw walnuts, pumpkin seeds and hemp seeds. The best source of omega 9 is cold-pressed extra virgin olive oil.

Fighting those free radicals

One more thing about fats. They are very labile, breaking down quickly when exposed to air, heat or light. When they do, they oxidize, rancidify and produce free radicals. Free radicals weren't very popular in the '60s, and we don't want them around now either. Free radicals are unstable molecules which damage cellular DNA and are implicated in the aging and cancerous process of every cell in the body. They are known culprits in Alzheimers and Parkinsons disease, and can probably be implicated in heart disease and most other human degenerative conditions. One way to minimize them is to avoid heating oils as much as possible. Some of the recipes in this book do contain heated oils, but it is best to keep the oils and the heating to a minimum. Including antioxidant-rich, radical-quenching ingredients in the recipes can really help.

Cavemen were smarter than you think

So back to our hunter-gatherers. Of course,

they didn't know much about food biochemistry, yet instinctively they ate a diet rich in the same phytonutrients (plant chemicals) that have become the buzzwords of modern nutritional research: antioxidants, bioflavonoids, sulforaphanes, indoles, lignans, isoflavones, carotenoids, enzymes, and chlorophyll, to name a few. There are actually over 12,000 phytonutrients in the plant kingdom.

Furthermore, the paleolithic diet was unadulterated: No xenobiotics (foreign chemical additives), no pesticides, no hormones, no bioengineering, no irradiation, no charbroiling, (God help us) no microwaving -- in fact, no stoves! Well, isn't the microwave good for anything? Absolutely! Put a big bow on it and give it to your worst enemy for Christmas!

2: Eat colorful

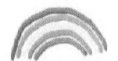 The second fundamental principle of healthy eating is EAT COLORFUL.

What color is the typical American diet? White! White flour, white sugar, white bread, white pasta, white milk, white cheese, white rice, white potatoes.... No color! White flour has one job, and you probably learned about it in first grade: to make paper mache! So if you want to glue your intestines together, keep eating the "glue-ten" in white flour. And cow's milk has one job: to turn a 50-pound calf into a 500-pound cow. I don't know about you, but that's not the figure I strive for. Do you know we are the only species that consumes another species' milk? That means we're right and the entire animal kingdom has got it wrong. Well, I find that "udder-ly" ridiculous!

A colorful cornucopia

So how does one get a colorful diet? By consuming loads of fruits and vegetables. There are literally tens of thousands of scientific studies demonstrating the importance of fruits and vegetables to human health. Researchers studying 600,000 Seventh-Day Adventists at the Loma Linda University School of Public Health, for example, observed longer than average lifespans with lower incidence of heart disease and cancer among the vegetarians raised on a heavy plant-based diet.

According to Richard DuBois, MD, Chief of Internal Medicine at Atlanta Medical Center and a top authority on infectious disease, over 4500 studies show that whole fruits and veggies specifically prevent cancer. Andrew Weil, MD, probably the most famous Harvard-trained physician practicing alternative medicine in the world, recently stated: "A diet high in fruits and vegetables is associated with a lower risk of 15 types of cancer, among them colon, breast, cervix, and lung."

A recent meta-analysis (a research study on the research studies) of 170 different studies from 17 different nations revealed that the people who eat the most fruits and vegetables have half the cancer rates of those who eat the least. And devouring fruits and vegetables is not only protective of cancer. It can also slash one's chances of heart attack, stroke, and hypertension, as well as a wide range of other disease conditions.

All vegetables are not equal

The "Five-a-Day" campaign of the US Department of Agriculture and the American Cancer Society is certainly a step in the right direction. Actually, one should strive to consume *double* that number of fist-sized servings of fresh fruits and vegetables daily — ideally three servings of fruit and six or seven of veggies. At this point, we had better define the term "vegetable." I recently had a patient lean over, look me in the eye, and ask, "What exactly do you mean by a *vegetable*?" That's kind of sad, but quite understandable, considering that the top three vegetables consumed in this country are catsup, iceberg lettuce, and French fries. The former was named a vegetable by the late President Ronald Reagan — probably the least valuable part of his legacy to this country. Iceberg lettuce is 99 percent water, with the remaining one percent hardly qualifying for green. And the brief life history of a French fry (which, by the way, is called "American fry" in France): In your mouth a few minutes, in your stomach a few hours, and on your hips for the rest of your life!

The mighty carotenes

Back to the issue of colors. Fruits and

vegetables get their colors from carotenoids, a large group of 600 or so natural plant chemicals. Many of us have heard of beta-carotene, but that is one of the weakest of the carotenes. And we want the full spectrum of carotenes as they are found in whole foods, not just in fractionated supplements. Furthermore, carotenes are found not only in carrots, not only in orange fruits and vegetables, but also in fresh produce that is yellow, red, purple and green.

Carotenes play two enormous roles in our health. First, they boost immune function. There are hundreds of studies on file with the National Cancer Institute demonstrating that carotenes can activate T-cells, natural killer cells, and macrophages, all key players in our immune system. Secondly, carotenes are powerful antioxidants, essential for quenching free radicals. One well-known carotene is lycopene, found in red foods like tomatoes and beets, which packs a nutritional punch against prostate cancer, for example.

Fabulous fiber

Besides carotenes, fruits and vegetables are also rich in fiber. Fiber is the non-nutritive part of whole foods like beans, legumes, seeds, nuts, whole grains, fruits and vegetables. It can bind up and escort out cancer-promoting hormones and chemicals. Ideally, we should be consuming about 50 grams of fiber daily, whereas the typical American diet contains less than five grams of fiber.

Low fiber has been connected to colon cancer, breast cancer, prostate cancer, lymphatic cancer, and probably a whole range of other cancers. It is just as likely to be a factor in cardiovascular disease and diabetes, as well as other chronic health problems. The more fiber we consume, the more frequent and bulky are our solid eliminations through the bowel. As Dr. Dennis Burkitt wisely observed, "Small stools, large hospitals."

It's easy being green

The one color God put on this planet more than any other is the color green. Chlorophyll is one of the most powerful wound-healers and blood-builders known. Its molecular structure is nearly identical to that of hemoglobin, with the exception that the iron atom is replaced by magnesium. We should be consuming vegetables that are as dark green as possible every day. They are actually higher in bioavailable calcium than dairy products, with a perfect ratio of calcium and magnesium.

Craving crucifers

One more important group of phytonutrients can be found in the cruciferous or brassica family of vegetables, which includes broccoli, cauliflower, cabbage, kale, collard and brussels sprouts. These foods have many anti-cancer properties. This is mainly due to their content of indole and sulfur compounds, which support key liver enzyme functions and detoxification pathways that can neutralize dangerous hormones and carcinogens. In an experiment conducted in Israel, women living in a farm community were placed on a diet high in crucifers. In only seven days, the dangerous estrogen that promotes breast cancer was converted into a benign form of estrogen.

3: Eat Alkaline

A third healthy-eating fundamental is EAT ALKALINE.

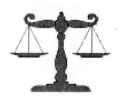

Acid-alkaline balance is a key principle often ignored even by those who habitually eat "health foods." Many researchers are encouraging consumption of a dietary ratio of about 80 percent plant-based foods to 20 percent animal foods. That correlates roughly with an 80 percent alkaline and a 20 percent acid diet.

Dr. William Howard Hay, a physician who wrote a book at the turn of the last century called *How to Always Be Well*, stressed that very same ratio. The body starts to heal, he stated, when its intracellular pH (potential Hydrogen, a measure of acidity) is at about 7.3, which is slightly on the alkaline side. If we think of a scale from 0 to 14, with 0 being the most acid and 14 being the most alkaline, then 7 would be neutral, about the pH of water. At the extremes of acidosis or alkalosis, we cannot survive, but at the optimal level of 7.3 or 7.4 we thrive. Tumor cells — and most diseases — thrive in acidosis. Because one of the best ways of maintaining appropriate pH is to eat alkalizing foods, Dr. Hay, and many other experts to follow, urged that we consume about 80 percent of our diet from the alkaline group of foods, and only 20 percent of our diet from the acid group. As microbiologist Dr. Robert Young states in his book, *The pH Miracle*, "Striking the optimum 80/20 balance can result in dramatic weight loss, rebuilt stamina...and vibrant health."

When you dine, think alkaline

So which foods are which? Roughly speaking, all fresh fruits and vegetables are alkaline. (The more we cook them, the closer they move to the acid side.) Proteins (amino acids) like meat, fish, milk, eggs, and poultry are acidifying, as are fats, grains, pasta and sugars. This does not mean that we can never eat those foods; it means that ideally we consume them only as one-fifth of our total daily diet.

The typical American diet is highly acidic. Our typical breakfast — cereal and milk, bagel and coffee, bacon and eggs — is all acid. Our typical lunch — a sandwich of meat or cheese, a slice of pizza, hamburger on a bun, with maybe a token piece of lettuce — is also acidic. The same goes for the typical American dinner — meat and potatoes, spaghetti and meatballs, chicken and rice — perhaps a few stringbeans. Even those who are into health foods and choose whole grain with the skin removed, are still consuming a heavily acid meal.

Now, if the researchers and clinicians who talk about acid-alkaline balance are right — and the evidence says they are — and we are eating this way three meals a day, seven days a week, 365 days a year, decade after decade after decade, is it any wonder so many of us are sick?

4: Eat Organic

The fourth principle of healthy eating is EAT ORGANIC.

Now, to most of us, organic produce is that which is grown without chemical pesticides or other carcinogenic and mutagenic additives. This is certainly desirable and protective of our health. But what is not usually realized is that organic produce means more than what is left *out*; it means especially what is left *in* — specifically minerals. Plants absorb close to 70 nutrients from the soil, but ordinary fertilizers only provide a few.

Organic farmers see to it that the trace minerals are plowed back into the soil through composting and that crops are rotated so that the same crop does not deplete the same minerals from the same soil every year. Often these farmers use the Biblical concept of letting the land lie fallow, so that it can replenish its mineral stores. The result is an abundance of minerals that are lacking in non-organic produce.

Several years ago, the Rutgers University School of Agriculture issued the Firman Baer report, comparing the mineral content of organically grown vegetables with that of non-organic vegetables. The figures are telling. The calcium content of cabbage, for example, was 60 parts per million in the organically-grown cabbage, versus only 17.5 parts per million in the inorganic cabbage. Similarly, the magnesium content of organic snap beans was 60 parts per million, whereas the magnesium content of non-organic snap beans was 14.8. Looking at the potassium content of lettuce, the organic lettuce contained 176.5 parts per million, while the inorganic lettuce contained only 53.7. The differences in iron content were most marked: In the organically grown tomatoes, 1938 parts; in the non-organic tomatoes, one!

Vegetable	Mineral	Organic	Non-organic
Cabbage	Calcium	60	17.5
Snap beans	Magnesium	60	14.8
Lettuce	Potassium	176.5	53.7
Tomatoes	Iron	1938	1

Mineral content in parts per million

So to reiterate, the best diets all have in common these four basic principles:

- ♦ EAT PRIMITIVE
- ♦ EAT COLORFUL
- ♦ EAT ALKALINE
- ♦ EAT ORGANIC.

According to the doctors and other health experts whose words I quote on nearly every page of this book, adhering to these guidelines will help you prevent cancer, heart disease, diabetes, and a broad range of illnesses; they will help you maintain a healthy weight; and they will help you feel vibrantly alive well into your golden years.

APPETIZERS & SNACKS

Apple Walnut Canapes

1 C walnuts
2 red apples, cored and quartered, skin left on
1 can water chestnuts (8 oz), drained
1/4 C honey
3 large zucchini

Slice zucchini on the diagonal, to form oval slices
1/4 inch thick. Pulse process together walnuts,
apples, water chestnuts and honey to a coarse
blend. Spread on zucchini slices.

Yield: 24-30 canapes

NUTRI-NOTE:
Zucchini is rich in
organic sodium,
an alkaline
element that
helps to
neutralize acid
and restore a
sodium-
exhausted liver.

*"'We are what we eat...' is probably the
...most important statement ever made
concerning the health of the human race."*

John H. Tobe

Artichoke Appetizer

1 T olive oil
1 large onion, thinly sliced
2 medium cloves garlic, minced
14 oz can artichoke hearts packed in water,
    drained and quartered
1 T lemon juice
4 leaves Boston lettuce

In a large skillet, saute onion in oil over low heat, stirring occasionally, for 1 minute or until golden brown. Add garlic and cook 1 minute more. Stir in artichoke hearts and lemon juice. Cover and simmer for 5 minutes. Serve warm over lettuce leaf.

Yield: 4 servings

NUTRI-NOTE: Garlic has a strengthening, laxative effect, relieves indigestion, disinfects the stomach, kills bacteria in the large intestine, and neutralizes poisons.

"Man's place in future history will depend in no small degree on the food he eats."

Dr. James McLester

Artichoke Dip

14 oz can artichoke hearts, packed in water,
   drained
5 oz goat cheese, softened
1/2 C vanilla yogurt
1 scallion, thinly sliced
2 tsp finely minced garlic
2 tsp lemon juice
sea salt to taste
pepper to taste
dash paprika

Pulse process together artichokes, cheese,
yogurt, and lemon juice. Stir in garlic, seasonings
and scallion.

Yield: Approximately 2 cups

TASTY TIP:
Serve with
vegetable
crudites or
sprouted grain
bread.

*"Ninety percent of all conditions other than...
contagious disease and...physical injuries
are directly traceable to diet."*

Sir William Osler, MD

Artichokes with Dijon Aioli

3 whole globe artichoke heads
1 egg yolk
2 tsp hot water
1/4 C pine nuts
1 T Dijon mustard
1 T extra virgin olive oil
1 clove garlic, minced
2 tsp lemon juice
1/2 tsp sea salt

Wash artichokes, cut off stem and discard discolored outer leaves. Clip off 1 inch of top. Place in boiling water to cover, with 1 tsp lemon juice and sea salt. Simmer 30 minutes. In a blender, combine remaining lemon juice, egg, water, mustard, garlic, and pine nuts. Blend at low speed. While blender is running, drizzle oil through hole in top. Serve artichokes with sauce in separate, individual dishes.

Yield: 3 servings

NUTRI-NOTE:
Artichokes help lower cholesterol and blood sugar and stimulate bile flow.

"Food is a powerful medicine, probably the most powerful medicine you will ever take."

Dr. Cass Ingram

Banana Nut Bread

1 C raw walnuts
1 1/3 C whole wheat flour
2 T arrowroot
1 T Sucanat
1/2 tsp cinnamon
2 tsp baking soda
1 1/2 C very ripe bananas (about 2), mashed
1/4 C unsweetened applesauce
1/4 C honey
2 eggs
1 tsp vanilla
1 tsp walnut oil

Preheat oven to 325 F. Lightly grease a 9 by 5 inch loaf pan with walnut oil. Grind 1/4 C nuts in processor to a fine powder. Place in large mixing bowl. Sift together flour, arrowroot, and baking soda into bowl and mix well with walnut meal. Coarse chop remaining nuts and add to dry ingredients. Combine eggs, bananas, applesauce honey and vanilla in blender. Pour liquid mixture into dry mixture and stir gently to mix. Pour into loaf pan, cover loosely with foil, and bake for 55 minutes or until toothpick inserted in center comes out clean. After 10 minutes at room temperature, turn loaf out on wire rack to cool.

Yield: 8 thick slices

"If you can't change your cooking and eating for six months, you're not ready to get well."

Sherry Rogers, MD

Basil Pesto

1/4 C olive oil
5 cloves garlic, chopped
1/2 C pine nuts
2 C fresh basil
1/4 C lemon juice
1 tsp sea salt

Blend all ingredients thoroughly in a blender. Serve with sunflower crackers or sprouted grain bread.

Yield: About 1 cup

TASTY TIP:
This yummy, filling pesto can also be served as a sauce for wraps, chicken, or pasta.

"A mountain of research has shown that food plays an important role in cancer of the breast, colon, prostate, and other organs, and can increase or decrease the likelihood of survival of cancer patients."

Neal Barnard, MD

Belgian Endive Boats

3 C raw pecans
16 Deglet Noor dates, pitted
1/4 C lemon juice
20 outer leaves Belgian endive

Wash endive leaves, pat dry and set aside.
Process remaining ingredients in processor until
finely chopped. Stuff each endive leaf with nut
mixture. Chill and serve — wonderfully filling!

Yield: 20 generous hors d'oeuvre

*"Father technology has not brought us freedom
from disease...because we have been dazzled by
his stepchildren – fast foods, fractionated foods,
convenience foods, packaged foods, fake foods,
embalmed foods, ersatz foods...."*

Sally Fallon

Black Bean Dip

1 can (15 oz) black beans, rinsed and drained
1/4 C diced onion
1/8 tsp salt
2 T vegetable broth
1/2 tsp ground cumin
2 T raw tahini
2 medium cloves garlic, minced
2 T lemon juice
cayenne to taste (optional)

In a food processor, combine all ingredients. Refrigerate 1-2 hours for flavors to blend. Serve with pita triangles or mini carrots and celery chunks.

Yield: 12 ounces

NUTRI-NOTE: One cup of cooked beans per day can significantly lower cholesterol, reduce cancer risk, and improve bowel function.

"The doctor of the future will give no medicine, but will interest his patients in the cure of the human frame, in diet and in the cause and prevention of disease."

Thomas A. Edison

Carrot Flax Muffins

1 C freshly ground flaxseeds
7/8 C millet flour
1 tsp baking powder (aluminum-free)
1 tsp baking soda
1/3 C maple syrup
1/2 C water
1/2 C unsweetened applesauce
1/4 C walnut oil
2/3 C grated carrots
1 tsp allspice

Preheat oven to 375 F. Combine maple syrup, water, applesauce, oil and carrots. In a separate bowl, combine remaining ingredients well. Stir into wet ingredients. Spoon batter into oiled muffin tin. Bake for 25 minutes or until toothpick inserted into muffin center comes out clean. Cool on rack.

Yield: 8 muffins

NUTRI-NOTE: In a recent University of Toronto study of women due for breast cancer surgery, tumor size reduced after only one month on daily flaxseed muffins.

*"The dietician of today
will be the doctor of tomorrow."*

Dr. Alexis Carrel

Celery Boats with Bean Dip

4 C cooked white beans, drained
2 cloves garlic, minced
1/4 C lemon juice
2 tsp extra virgin olive oil
1 tsp finely chopped fresh or 1/2 tsp dried parsley
sea salt to taste
pepper to taste
5 stalks of celery, cut into bite-sized pieces

Put all ingredients except parsley into food processor and blend until creamy. Chill. Scoop into celery slices and garnish with parsley.

Yield: 5 servings

NUTRI-NOTE:
Olive oil makes cells less prone to free radical damage, helping to protect them from aging and cancer.

"Eat to live, do not merely live to eat."

Benjamin Franklin

Guacamole

3 large ripe avocados
1 tsp sea salt
1/4 C lemon juice
3 cloves garlic
1 small tomato, finely chopped
1/2 medium onion, finely chopped

Blend avocados, salt, lemon juice and garlic in a food processor until creamy. Mix in a bowl with the chopped ingredients. Serve chilled over bed of Boston lettuce with corn chips.

Yield: 4-6 servings

TASTY TIP:
Use 1 red bell pepper, finely chopped instead of tomato.

"And God said: 'Behold, I have given you every herb yielding seed, which is upon the face of all the earth, and every tree in which is the fruit of a tree yielding seed – to you it shall be for food.'"

Genesis 1:29

Hazelnut Rollups

1/2 C hazelnuts
1/4 C sunflower seeds
1/4 C finely chopped celery
2 T diced sweet red pepper
2 tsp Sucanat
1 T water
2 T parsley flakes
2 T finely chopped onion
1 1/2 tsp lemon juice
10 leaves Boston, bibb or butterhead lettuce,
    about 4 inches square

Coarsely chop nuts and seeds in food processor using the S blade. Add remaining ingredients and pulse chop until well mixed but not pasty. Wash lettuce leaves and pat dry. Place about 1 heaping T of mixture into center of each lettuce leaf. Roll tightly, parallel to leaf spine, into cones, allowing curled ends of leaf to flair. Fasten with toothpicks. Arrange on serving platter fan side out.

Yield: 10 rollups

NUTRI-NOTE:
Raw sunflower seeds are an excellent source of zinc, protective against prostate cancer.

"The roots of cancer arise from metabolic dysfunction – and metabolic dysfunction is directly influenced by diet."

Mauris Emeka

Hummus-Tahini

1 can (15 oz) chickpeas (garbanzo beans)
3 T raw sesame tahini
1 T extra virgin olive oil
1 1/2 cloves garlic, diced
1/4 tsp sea salt
dash ground cumin (optional)
dash cayenne (optional)
3 T lemon juice
2 T water
1/2 T fresh parsley, chopped
pinch paprika

Drain and rinse chickpeas. In food processor, combine all ingredients except parsley and paprika. Process until smooth and creamy. Place in serving bowl and sprinkle with parsley and paprika. Chill before serving.

Yield: 1 2/3 cups

TASTY TIP:
Serve with whole wheat pita triangles or with cut raw vegetables.

*"It is just as easy to eat right
as it is to eat wrong."*

Dr. Cass Ingram

Lentil Mushroom Hors d'Oeuvre

2 C cooked green lentils, mashed
2 scallions, minced
1 small onion, minced
2 tsp extra virgin olive oil
1/4 tsp dried oregano
1/4 tsp dried thyme
dash pepper to taste
sea salt to taste
16 large white mushrooms

Preheat oven to 450 degrees F. Saute scallion and onion in oil over medium heat for 3 minutes. Add lentils, salt and spices and saute over low heat 3 minutes more. Remove from heat. Remove stems from mushrooms. Stuff mushrooms with lentil mixture. Place on lightly oiled pan and bake 12 minutes. Serve warm.

Yield: 16 hors d'oeuvre

NUTRI-NOTE:
Lentils contain nitrilosides, food factors which, combined with enzymes found only in cancer cells, produce compounds poisonous to those cells.

"The largely new dietary pattern adopted... within the past one hundred years appears to go beyond what our genes can tolerate."

Drs. S. Boyd Eaton and Melvin Konner

Mushroom Chickpea Pate

1 lb button mushrooms, washed and sliced
1 medium onion, chopped
2 large cloves garlic, minced
1 T extra virgin olive oil
1 can (15 oz) chickpeas, rinsed and drained
1 C hazelnuts or pecans, coarsely ground
1 T Sucanat
1 tsp Mrs. Dash seasoning
1/2 tsp sea salt
1/4 tsp paprika

Quickly mash chickpeas in processor for 10 seconds. Place into large bowl and stir in nuts, Sucanat and seasonings. In large frypan, saute onions and mushrooms in olive oil over medium heat for 5 minutes. Add garlic and cook 2 more minutes. Process sauteed mixture until creamy. Add to chickpea mixture and stir until well incorporated. Chill. Serve with celery chunks.

Yield: 2 cups

TASTY TIP:
Pates may also be stuffed into mushroom caps, scooped onto Boston lettuce leaves, or spread on rice crackers, zucchini slices, or triangles of sprouted grain bread.

*"Leave thy drugs in the chemist's pot
if thou can heal the patient with food."*

Hippocrates

No-Grain Bread Muffins

1 C flaxseeds, finely ground
1 C walnuts, chopped
3/4 C whey protein powder
4 T Sucanat
2 tsp baking powder (aluminum-free)
1 tsp baking soda
1 1/2 tsp cinnamon
1/4 tsp salt
4 tsp walnut oil
2 eggs, beaten
2 tsp vanilla
2/3 C zucchini, peeled and grated
2/3 C ricotta cheese

Preheat oven to 350 F. In a small bowl, mix flax, protein powder, Sucanat, baking powder, baking soda, cinnamon and salt. In a large bowl, mix oil, eggs, vanilla, grated zucchini, and cheese. Fold dry ingredients into liquid ingredients. Fold walnuts into mixture. Push by spoonfuls into muffin tins and bake for 20 minutes. Let cool and serve with unsweetened preserves or apple butter. Refrigerate unused muffins.

Yield: 12 muffins

HELPFUL HINT:
Lining the muffin tin with paper muffin cups makes muffin removal and tin cleanup a breeze!

"If the body is nourished correctly, it usually is not vulnerable to disease."

William Howard Hay, MD

Nut Stuffed Celery

2 large celery stalks, leaves removed
4 T almond butter
2 T ground flaxseeds
2 T sunflower seeds, ground
1/8 tsp sea salt
dash lemon juice (optional)

Rinse and dry celery and cut into 2 inch pieces.
Mix together remaining ingredients. Add lemon
juice if thinning is needed. Stuff into celery. Chill
before serving.

Yield: Approximately 12 pieces

HELPFUL HINT:
Use raw almond
butter if possible.
Make sure it is
well
homogenized
before mixing
with other
ingredients.

*"The average person uses more care
in selecting the grade of gasoline to put
into their automobiles than they do
the food they put in their mouth."*

Rev . George Malkmus

Ratatouille Provencal

1/3 C extra virgin olive oil
1 large onion, thinly sliced
1 eggplant, cut into small pieces
1 green pepper, thinly sliced
2 tomatoes, peeled and sliced
2 cloves garlic, minced
3/4 tsp sea salt
1/4 tsp dried basil

In a large fry pan, heat the oil over medium-low heat. Add sliced onion and cook for 10 minutes, stirring occasionally. Add eggplant and green pepper. Cover and cook for 10 minutes. Periodically lift cover to stir. If vegetables begin to stick to bottom, add a few drops of water. Add tomatoes, garlic, salt and basil and cook for 10 more minutes. Serve on lettuce leaf with pita triangles.

Yield: 6 servings

NUTRI-NOTE:
Eggplants, tomatoes, peppers (and white potatoes) are members of the nightshade family. They should be avoided by those with arthritic tendencies.

"The risks of common forms of cancer are reduced by 50 percent in countries where about a pound of fruits and vegetables is eaten each day."

David Heber, MD, PhD

Spinach Goat Cheese Spread

4 oz goat cheese, softened
2 C fresh baby spinach leaves
1 scallion, chopped
1/4 stalk celery, coarsely chopped
1 clove garlic, diced
1 tsp lemon juice
1 T raw pine nuts
sea salt to taste

Using S blade of food processor, combine
spinach, scallion, celery, garlic, and lemon juice.
Add pine nuts and pulse until coarsely included.
Place in serving bowl and stir in cheese.   Season
to taste with salt. Refrigerate several hours
before serving with crackers.

Yield: 6 ounces

NUTRI-NOTE:
Goat cheese is
much more
digestible in the
human body than
cow's milk
cheese.

*"The most common disease-producing
factors are from food deficiencies
[and] errors in diet."*

D. T. Quigley, MD

Stuffed Mushrooms

8 large fresh stuffing mushrooms
1/4 C matzo meal
2 T chopped walnuts
2 tsp dry chopped chives
1 tsp dry parsley flakes
1/2 tsp paprika
1/2 tsp sea salt or Herbamare
1/4 tsp pepper
2 T almond milk
1 T goat cheese
1 tsp honey
1 T olive oil

Preheat oven to 400 F. Wash mushrooms and pat dry. Carefully snap off stems from caps and chop coarsely. In processor, combine mushroom stems, matzo meal, walnuts, chives, parsley, paprika, salt, pepper, almond milk, cheese, and honey until well blended. Stuff caps. Grease bottom of 9 inch square pan with olive oil. Bake 20 minutes until caps are just tender and tops are slightly browned. Serve hot.

Yield: 8 mushrooms

*"Food values can be measured
only in terms of health —
not by their cost per pound."*

Dr. R. G. Jackson

Sunflower Crackers

1 C sunflower seeds
1/2 C shredded unsweetened coconut
1/4 C cold water
1/4 tsp sea salt
olive oil natural cooking spray

In a food processor, combine seeds, coconut, salt and water until pasty. Lightly spray a brownie pan (about 9 by 7 by 1 inch) with cooking spray. Flatten out dough and press into pan evenly to edges. Score with knife into squares. Place in cold oven. Turn on oven to 300 F and bake 12 minutes. Cool 5 minutes. Carefully break apart crackers.

Yield: 20-24 crackers

TASTY TIP:
Serve crackers with pesto, pate, or spread.

"Cancer is the final stage in years of acting against the laws of nature."

Helmut Wandmaker

Vegetable Sushi Rolls

1/2 C short grain brown rice, rinsed well
3/4 C water
2 T rice wine vinegar
1/2 C almond butter, stirred well
2 sheets nori
1 avocado, peeled and sliced thinly lengthwise
1/2 cucumber, peeled, seeded, cut thinly
    lengthwise
2 carrots, julienned in thin strips

Place rice and water in medium saucepan. Cover,
bring to boil, then reduce heat to low and cook for 25
minutes. Remove from heat and leave covered for
another 10 minutes. Transfer rice to mixing bowl. Pour
vinegar evenly over rice. Cover with moist towel to
prevent surface from drying. Spread almond butter
evenly over nori sheets. Place rice in center of nori
and spread to all four corners. Place avocado,
cucumber, and carrots over rice about 1 inch from
sides. Roll the nori tghtly, pushing in the rice and
vegetables that are sticking out of the ends. Wet a
knife and slice the rolls in half, then in thirds.

Yield: 12 pieces

NUTRI-NOTE:
Nori has
demonstrated anti-
ulcer and anti-
microbial effects.

*"[Cancer] is caused by poisons created
in our bodies by the food we eat."*

Sir William A. Lane, MD

Veggie Crudites with Honey Mustard Sauce

1 C mini carrots
1 C raw cauliflower florets
1 C raw broccoli florets
1 red pepper, cut into bite-sized pieces
1 medium zucchini, cut into bite-sized chunks
1/4 C water
1/4 C honey
2 T plus 2 tsp Dijon mustard
1 C raw cashews

In a coffee mill, grind cashews to a very fine powder. In a blender, combine water, honey, mustard and cashews until well blended. Spoon dip into small serving bowl placed in center of serving tray. Arrange vegetables around dip. Serve chilled.

Yield: About 4 servings

NUTRI-NOTE: Broccoli, a member of the cancer-protective cruciferous family, is also high in calcium and vitamin C.

"Colorize your diet."

David Heber, MD, PhD

Walnut Onion Pate

1 C walnuts
1/4 C pine nuts
1/2 C finely chopped onions
1/2 stalk celery, chopped
1/2 T extra virgin olive oil
1 T dried basil
1/4 tsp paprika
1/4 tsp dried basil
1 tsp honey
2 T water

Process all with S blade to make a creamy pate. Garnish with a dash of paprika. Chill about 2 hours. Stuff in celery chunks or serve with rice crackers.

Yield: 1 1/3 cups

NUTRI-NOTE:
Half a raw onion per day can boost good HDL blood cholesterol by thirty percent.

"Americans don't have vitamin deficiencies -- we have whole food deficiencies."

Delia Garcia, MD

Wilted Frisee with Shitake

4 tsp extra virgin olive oil
2 T minced shallots
1 C thinly sliced shitake mushrooms
4 C curly endive
1 tsp balsamic vinegar
dash sea salt

Heat olive oil in a large skillet over medium heat.
Add shallots and mushrooms and cook 2 minutes,
stirring frequently. Add curly endive and cook 1
minute longer, until greens wilt. Remove from
heat and drizzle with balsamic vinegar. Add salt
to taste.

Yield: 2 servings

*"There is a natural affinitybetween
natural foods and the human body.
They share the earth as a source,
and the body so fed holds energies to be
found in no other way. We call it health."*

Pearl S. Buck

SOUPS & BROTHS

Alkaline Broth

1 C celery, diced (2 large stalks)
1 C green beans, diced (about 1/4 lb)
1 C zucchini, diced (1 small squash)
1 C sweet potato or yam, diced
1 clove garlic, minced
1/2 small onion
6 C water

Place all vegetables and water in large pot and bring to boil for 3 minutes. Cover and simmer vegetables for 25-30 minutes. Strain vegetables and discard.

Yield: 6 cups

NUTRI-NOTE: Drink 1 cup of broth twice daily, about 10 a.m. and 4 p.m. This broth is heavily laden with minerals and will help eliminate excess acidity.

"Alkaline foods are most valuable for the sick person."

Dr. Bernard Jensen

Beet Borsht

1 medium beet, peeled and chopped
1/4 C raw almond butter
1/4 C onion, diced
1/2 stalk celery, chopped
1/4 tsp sea salt
1/2 tsp honey
1 C water
2 heaping T vanilla yogurt

Blend all ingredients except yogurt until creamy.
Chill and serve with a dollop of yogurt on top.

Yield: 2 servings

NUTRI-NOTE:
Raw beets fight
cancer and are,
like tomatoes, a
rich source of
the antioxidant
lycopene.

"God has prescribed whole, natural foods."

Fred Miller, DDS

Black Bean Soup

1 T extra virgin olive oil
4 cloves garlic, diced
1 small red onion, chopped
1 tsp cumin
4 cans seasoned black beans (15 oz each)
6 C chicken stock or vegetable stock
pepper to taste
sea salt to taste

Saute onions in oil over medium heat until translucent. Add garlic and cook another minute. Place into soup pot. Add all of the other ingredients. Simmer, covered, for about 30 minutes.

Yield: 8 cups

NUTRI-NOTE:
Beans help to control insulin and blood sugar.

"Food eaten today is about as far removed from the natural diet of man as man is from his primitive jungle. Man, however, still has approximately the same digestive apparatus ...as his remote ancestors."

Henry Biehler, MD

Carrot Avocado Soup

2 C fresh carrot juice (8-10 large carrots)
2 avocados
1/2 tsp ground cumin
2 tsp lemon juice
1/2 tsp vanilla extract
1/4 C fresh apple juice
1/2 C sprouts
pinch sea salt
dash allspice

In a blender, combine the carrot juice and avocado. Add the lemon juice, vanilla, apple juice, salt and spices and blend again. Garnish with sprouts and serve cold.

Yield: 3-4 servings

"Of the ten million red blood cells built every second by the body, not a single one was ever built from the slogan on a package."

Henry Trautmann, MD

Chicken Escarole Soup

6 C chicken broth or vegetable broth
2 T tomato paste
2 tsp sea salt
dash pepper
1 large onion, chopped
1 carrot, chopped
1 C diced celery
4 C shredded escarole
2 C diced cooked chicken

Mix all ingredients together in a soup pot. Bring to a boil, then simmer, covered, for 30 minutes.

Yield: 8 cups

"I have made no effort to determine the number of diseases which are directly dependent upon diet, but I believe I would not be far out of the way if I should say every disease to which man is heir."

Dr. Harvey Wiley

Chilled Cantaloupe Soup

1 ripe cantaloupe
3/4 C fresh orange juice
1/2 tsp vanilla
1/2 tsp maple syrup (optional)
2 mint leaves

Cut cantaloupe at the equator. Remove seeds
from each half and discard. Scoop out most of
the melon, taking care not to cut into green flesh,
and puree in blender with orange juice and
vanilla. Chill melon and blended juice for about 3
hours. Pour liquid into melon halves and garnish
with mint leaves.

Yield: 2 servings

NUTRI-NOTE:
To level melon bowls
that lean, carefully slice
off a very thin layer of
bottom rind from the
uneven side, or perch
atop small dessert bowl
base.

*"Every morsel of food that goes into your body helps
or hurts you. When it is a live, natural food, it
becomes part of your blood [and] bathes every cell
in your body.... When that morsel is not a live food,
but an artificial, synthetic, processed, canned or
embalmed food, it has to be expelled at great cost...."*

Dr. Bernard Jensen

Cream of Asparagus Soup

3 C asparagus, chopped
1 C raw cashews
1 tsp walnut oil
2 medium ripe avocados, peeled and pitted
1 clove garlic, minced
3 C water
1/4 C lemon juice
1 1/2 tsp honey
1 1/4 C vegetable broth
2 tsp Mrs. Dash table blend, ground
2 T fresh parsley, chopped
pinch sea salt
pepper to taste
6 fresh parsley sprigs

Steam asparagus about 5 minutes or until tender. In food processor, process cashews until butter starts sticking to sides. While processing, pour walnut oil, 1/2 tsp at a time, to produce a homo-homogenized thick ball. In a blender, combine avocados, 1 C asparagus, garlic, water, lemon juice, honey, cashew butter, and vegetable broth until smooth. Add parsley and seasonings and blend one minute more. Pour into pot with remaining chopped asparagus. Warm over medium heat, stirring frequently. Garnish with parsley.

Yield: 7 cups

"A proper diet can best restore the ill person to health without the necessity of employing drugs or questionable surgery."

Henry Biehler, MD

Cream of Mushroom Soup

1 C water
1/2 C almond butter
3 C white mushrooms, quartered
2 tsp maple syrup
pinch sea salt
dash pepper
3 T mushrooms, finely chopped

In a blender, combine the water and almond butter and blend. Add the quartered mushrooms, maple syrup, salt and pepper. Blend until smooth. Pour into individual bowls and top with the chopped mushrooms.

Yield: 2-3 servings

TASTY TIP:
Soup may also be served warm. Heat slowly, stirring constantly, to comfortable temperature. DO NOT BOIL.

"The United States leads the civilized world in chemicalized food and in degenerative diseases....The only possible explanation... is that the food, though the most abundant, is also the most unwholesome."

Dr. Franklin Bicknell

Creamy Avocado Soup

1/4 C raw cashews
4 medium ripe avocados, peeled and pitted
1 clove garlic, minced
3 C water
1/2 C lemon juice
1/2 tsp sea salt
1/4 tsp pepper
4 sprigs fresh parsley

Using food processor, blend cashews with 1/2 C water until smooth. Add avocados, garlic, lemon juice, salt and pepper and process together, slowly adding remaining water until thoroughly blended. Pour into serving bowls. Garnish with fresh parsley. Chill and serve cold.

Yield: 4 servings

NUTRI-NOTE:
Avocados have beneficial fatty acids and are excellent sources of plant-based protein.

"Disease and cookery originated simultaneously."

Dr. Edward Howell

Creamy Cauliflower Soup

2/3 C water
2 T chopped onion
1 stalk celery, chopped
2 T honey
1/4 tsp sea salt
1 tsp extra virgin olive oil
1 medium head cauliflower, steamed
pepper to taste
1/2 tsp Chinese five spice

Place all ingredients in food processor and puree.
Pour into a saucepan and heat slowly over
medium heat to a comfortable temperature,
stirring continuously. Thin with a few drops of
water if desired. Garnish with a dash of Chinese
spice and serve.

Yield: 3-4 servings

TASTY TIP:
For a healthful
mashed potato
substitute, omit
water and onion.
Add a pat of
organic butter if
desired.

*"Heredity plays its part when we are born,
and from that point onward...the condition
of the body is the result of just what we have
eaten habitually throughout our whole life."*

William Howard Hay, MD

Curried Pumpkin Soup

1 can (15 oz) unsweetened pumpkin
1 apple, peeled and diced
1 C apple juice
1/2 C vegetable stock
1 C water
1/2 medium onion, diced
1 tsp curry powder
1/4 tsp thyme
2 T honey
1/2 tsp parsley
1/8 tsp sea salt
1/8 tsp black pepper
1/4 tsp nutmeg

Place all ingredients except parsley in blender and blend thoroughly. Pour into large saucepan and simmer for 10 minutes, stirring frequently. Pour into bowls, garnish with parsley and serve.

Yield: 5 servings

NUTRI-NOTE: Turmeric (the main ingredient in curry) can inhibit the growth of stomach and breast tumors.

"We are all dietetic sinners; only a small percent of what we eat nourishes us; the balance goes to waste and loss of energy."

Sir William Osler

Escarole Bean Soup

1 lb escarole
2 1/2 C water
1 onion, chopped
2 cloves garlic, minced
1 C cooked white beans, navy or pinto beans
Mrs. Dash's seasonings to taste

Tear escarole into small pieces and wash thoroughly. Place in 5 qt soup pot and saute in 1/2 C water until bright green and just wilted. Set aside. In large saucepan, place remaining water, onion, and garlic and cook, covered, on low setting for 20 minutes. Add onion-garlic mixture to escarole. Stir in beans and seasonings and simmer, covered, approximately 10 minutes.

Yield: 4 servings

NUTRI-NOTE:
This filling soup has lots of fiber and no fat.

*"Most of what we eat is superfluous....
we only live off a quarter of all we swallow:
Doctors live off the other three quarters."*

Ancient Egyptian inscription

Gazpacho

1/2 C water
1/2 C extra virgin olive oil
4 large ripe tomatoes
2 large cloves garlic
1 T honey
1/4 C lemon juice
1 tsp sea salt
1 tsp dried or 1 bunch fresh basil
1 medium green bell pepper
1 small cucumber
1 small onion
1 T finely chopped parsley

Chop pepper, cucumber and onion into 1/4 inch pieces and set aside. Place remaining ingredients, except for parsley, in a blender or processor and blend until smooth. Pour blended mixture into two bowls and spoon in chopped vegetables. Garnish with chopped parsley. Chill and serve.

Yield: 2 servings

"Practically all disease succumbs to raw food."

John H. Tobe

Lentil Soup

3 C vegetable stock
2 C water
1 C dried green lentils
1/2 onion, chopped
1 large carrot, sliced
1/2 C chopped celery
2 cloves garlic, minced
2 bay leaves
1/2 tsp oregano
1/2 T extra virgin olive oil
1 T apple cider vinegar
1 tsp sea salt
14 oz can crushed tomatoes
1/4 tsp pepper

In a large soup pot, saute onion, carrot, celery and garlic in oil over medium heat for 5 minutes, stirring occasionally. If vegetables stick to pan, add a few drops of water. Pour in the stock and water and bring soup to a boil. Rinse lentils and add to boiling stock. Add all remaining ingredients. Reduce heat, cover, and simmer one hour or until lentils are very soft. Remove from heat and discard bay leaves.

Yield: 6 servings

HELPFUL HINT:
If soup is too thick, add water ½ C at a time.
For a creamier soup, puree half the soup in a blender, return to pot and reheat.

"A rich man can only be healthy if he eats as though he were poor."

John H. Tobe

Orange Almond Soup

1 1/4 C raw almonds
2 T unsalted butter
1/2 C chopped onion
1/2 tsp sea salt
1 1/2 C water
1 1/2 C fresh squeezed orange juice
1/2 tsp orange zest
dash pepper
dash mint flakes
1 orange, unpeeled

Soak almonds in water to cover for 8-12 hours. Rinse and drain. In a heavy skillet, sauté onions in butter over low heat, stirring, for 5 minutes or until onions are soft. Remove from heat. In a blender, puree almonds, onions, salt, orange zest, adding water and orange juice gradually until smooth. Pour into serving bowls. Slice off stem end of orange and cut into thin rounds. Place orange slices atop each bowl and garnish with mint flakes.

Yield: 4-5 servings

TASTY TIP:
This soup may also be served hot. Pour from blender into pot and heat gently without cooking. Pour into bowls, garnish, and serve immediately.

"You can't ignore the importance of good digestion. The joy of life...depends on a sound stomach."

Joseph Conrad

Raspberry Peach Soup

6 ripe peaches, peeled and pitted
1 C frozen raspberries
1 1/2 T lemon juice
2 1/4 C fresh apple juice
6 T raw almond butter
1 C water

Blend peaches with 1 C apple juice and lemon juice until pureed. Add almond butter, 1 C apple juice and 1 C water. Blend thoroughly. Pour into large pitcher and chill. Puree raspberries with 1/4 C apple juice. Pour soup into bowls and top with raspberry puree. Swirl through soup and serve cold.

Yield: 6 servings

"Every time that a natural substance is removed from a food, every time an adulterant is added to a food, the balance in nature is disturbed.... It took thousands of years for the body to adjust itself to changing environmental conditions. When these conditions are suddenly altered by the actions of men, the cells cannot make the adjustment — disease is the result."

Dr. Edward J. Ryan

Shitake Miso Soup

2 medium onions, peeled and sliced
7 C water
6 carrots, scrubbed and thinly sliced into pennies
2 kale leaves, washed and thinly sliced
6 fresh shitake mushrooms, stems removed
4 T red miso
2 sheets kelp or nori, cut into thin strips
2 scallions, thinly sliced

Place onions, kelp, and 6 C water in soup pot and bring to a boil. Simmer, covered, for 10 minutes. Add carrots and simmer for 5 more minutes. Add kale and simmer for 5 additional minutes. Thinly slice shitake mushrooms, add to soup, and simmer for one minute more. Turn off heat. Mix miso with one cup of water until dissolved and add to soup. Garnish with scallions and serve.

Yield: 8 servings

NUTRI-NOTE:
Do not heat soup once miso is added, or you will destroy valuable enzymes.

"How you feel – whether you sing, sigh or sob — is based mainly on how your fueling system works."

Henry Biehler, MD

Spinach Soup

1/2 T extra virgin olive oil
1/2 small onion, chopped
8 cloves garlic, diced
7 oz. jar roasted red peppers, sliced fine
12 oz fresh spinach, washed thoroughly
5 C vegetable or chicken stock
1/2 tsp sea salt
pepper to taste

Slowly saute onion and garlic in oil until translucent. Place into a soup pot. Add all of the other ingredients. Bring to a boil. Simmer, covered, about 30 minutes.

Yield: 6 servings

HELPFUL HINT:
You can substitute frozen chopped spinach, defrosted, for fresh spinach.

"If we were to use the knowledge about food which is now available to us, practically all sickness...would be wiped out in one generation."

Dr. Jonathan Forman

Strawberry Soup

10 ounce package fresh or frozen strawberries
2 tsp honey
1 tsp lemon juice
1 tsp almond extract
1 C vanilla whole yogurt
2 tsp maple syrup
6 ounces apple juice
fresh mint sprigs

Place strawberries in a blender or food processor. Add other ingredients in order listed and blend until very smooth. Chill before serving. Garnish with mint.

Yield: 4 servings

"The laws of nature are the laws of health, and he who lives according to these laws is never ill."

Leo W. Dowling

Summer Squash Soup

4 green or yellow squash, quartered
1 C sprouts
1 C fresh carrot juice
1 T walnut oil
1/4 tsp nutmeg
2 tsp diced onion
1 C almond milk

In a food processor, mix squash, carrot juice, almond milk, oil, onion and nutmeg until smooth. Garnish with sprouts. Serve cool.

Yield: 6 servings

NUTRI-NOTE: This soup is loaded with carotenes -- rich in powerful antioxidants and immune-boosters -- which the body converts to vitamin A as needed.

"No other single factor has so far-reaching and profound an influence on the maintenance of health as proper nutrition."

N. Philip Norman, MD

Tomato Soup

1 1/2 C fresh tomatoes, chopped
3 T tomato paste
3/4 C onion, chopped
1 stalk celery, chopped
3 T honey
1/2 tsp sea salt
1 tsp extra virgin olive oil
1/2 C water
1/4 tsp dried oregano

Place all ingredients into blender and puree until smooth.   Heat over medium heat, stirring frequently. Pour soup into serving bowls and garnish with dash of oregano.

Yield: 2 servings

HELPFUL HINT: For a short cut, 1 can (28 oz) crushed tomatoes may be used in place of other tomato ingredients. Thin with a few drops of water if desired.

"The unadulterated products of the good earth build up our health."

Ebba Waerland

Vegetable Puree

2 medium onions, chopped
2 stalks celery, chopped
2 T extra virgin olive oil
4 C vegetable broth
1 large yam, peeled and diced
2 parsnips, chopped
2 T fresh chopped parsley
dash sea salt
pinch black pepper
pinch dried marjoram

In a large soup pot, saute onions and celery in oil for 5 minutes over medium heat, stirring occasionally. Add broth, parsley, yams and parsnips. Simmer, covered, 10 minutes. Pour into blender with salt, pepper and marjoram and puree until smooth. Return to soup pot and simmer 3 minutes more.

Yield: 4-5 servings

"We're prisoners of our taste buds."

Harvey Diamond

Wild Mushroom Soup

2 T extra virgin olive oil
2 leeks, thinly sliced
8 oz assorted wild mushrooms (oyster, shitake, portobello, or chanterelle), sliced
1/2 C cooked wild rice
5 C vegetable stock
1 C canned tomatoes
1 tsp minced garlic clove
1 T dried chopped parsley
1 T dried chopped basil
1 tsp sea salt
1/4 tsp pepper

In a large soup pot, saute leeks in olive oil until soft. Add mushrooms and saute for about 3 minutes. Add stock, tomatoes, wild rice and garlic. Bring to a boil. Simmer 30 minutes, covered. Add parsley, basil, salt and pepper. Simmer another 5 minutes.

Yield: 7-8 servings

"Do not expect a program of correct eating to benefit you, if you are following it between meals."

Dr. R. A. Riggs

Winter Squash Soup

2 acorn squash, halved and seeded
2 butternut squash, halved and seeded
3 carrots, peeled and halved
1 large onion, thinly sliced
2 yams cut into quarters
2 apples, peeled, cored and halved
4 tsp curry powder (optional)
3/4 tsp ground ginger
3 T maple syrup
pinch of cayenne pepper
sea salt to taste
1 C apple juice
3 C vegetable stock
1/2 C pecans, finely chopped
1 apple, grated

Preheat oven to 350 F. Place squash halves skin side down in a large baking pan.   Place apples and all other vegetables in pan. Mix seasonings, syrup apple juice, and stock. Pour over vegetables. Cover with foil and bake for 2 hours or until vegetables are soft. Remove pan from oven and allow to cool slightly. Remove skins from apples, yams and squash. Puree in batches in a blender. Pour into large soup pot and heat slowly, stirring frequently. Garnish with grated apple and chopped pecans.

Yield: 4-6 servings

"The medical establishment still seems to believe that nutrition cannot prevent disease."

Julian Whitaker, MD

Zucchini Carrot Soup

1 medium zucchini, chopped
1 medium carrot, chopped
1/2 apple, grated
1 1/2 tsp minced scallion
1/4 tsp dry basil
1/2 clove garlic, minced (optional)
2 T raw tahini
1 1/4 C water
8 hazelnuts, ground

Set aside 2 T of the grated apple and the
hazelnuts. Blend all remaining ingredients
together until smooth. Pour into soup bowls.
Garnish with grated apple and hazelnuts. Chill
before serving.

Yield: 2 servings

*"Every day in America, more people die of diet-
related diseases than died in the terrorist attacks
...on September 11, 2001."*

M. Warren Peary

SALADS & DRESSINGS

Arugula Raspberry Salad

6 C baby arugula, rinsed and spun
1/2 C chopped walnuts
1/2 C goat cheese, flaked with a fork
1 C fresh raspberries

Place greens on chilled salad plates. Sprinkle goat cheese and walnuts over greens. Top with raspberries. Serve with Berry Dressing (see below).

Yield: 4 servings

"I am food. Head my plea:
I'll ruin you if you ruin me.
If you boil or fry my good away
You're the one that will have to pay!"

Dr. Henry Hudson

Asparagus Salad

1/2 C fresh asparagus, chopped in 1 inch pieces
1/4 C diced red pepper
1/4 C diced yellow pepper
1 T chopped fresh parsley
1 scallion, chopped
1/4 tsp orange zest
1/4 C orange juice
1/2 tsp lemon juice
1/4 tsp Herbamare or sea salt
1/2 T extra virgin olive oil

Mix together all ingredients. Let stand 1 hour.

Yield: 2 servings

HELPFUL HINT:
Break tough ends off asparagus spears before cutting. Eight thin spears will yield about one-half cup.

"Disease and cookery originated simultaneously."

Dr. Edward Howell

Baby Greens with Pears and Hazelnuts

2 ripe Bartlett pears
1/4 C fresh lemon juice
6 C baby spring greens, washed and spun dry
3/4 C sliced hazelnuts (filberts)

Peel, core, and cut the pears in thin wedges.
Toss in lemon juice, coating well to avoid
discoloration.   Place greens on salad plates,
arrange pear slices on greens, and sprinkle with
hazelnuts. Serve with Hazelnut Dijon dressing
(see below).

Yield: 4 servings

*"The greatest single factor in the production
of good health is the right kind of food –
and the greatest single factor in the production
of ill health is the wrong kind of food."*

Sir Robert McCarrison, MD

Berry Dressing

8 strawberries, tops removed
16-20 raspberries
2 T maple syrup
2 T extra virgin olive oil
2 T lemon juice
2 fresh basil leaves, chopped
sea salt to taste

In a blender, combine the berries, honey, oil, lemon juice, basil, and salt. Puree. Chill before serving.

Yield: 2-4 servings

*"If we eat wrongly, no doctor can cure us;
if we eat rightly, no doctor is needed."*

Dr. Victor Rocine

Carrot Ambrosia

2 C shredded carrots
1/2 C raisins
1/2 C shredded unsweetened coconut
5-6 leaves Boston lettuce
1/8 C olive oil
1 T lemon juice
3 T honey
1/4 C water

Shred carrots in food processor. Combine lemon juice, honey and water in a blender. With the motor still running, drizzle in olive oil a little at a time through the hole in the lid until dressing thickens. Mix carrots, coconut and raisins with dressing. Spoon onto lettuce leaves.

Yield: 5-6 servings

"Disease cannot live on good food."

John H. Tobe

Chickpea Salad

15-oz can chickpeas, drained and rinsed
1/2 C chopped red pepper
1 small red or sweet onion, diced
1 medium cucumber, chopped
1 T balsamic vinegar
2 T extra virgin olive oil
1/4 tsp garlic powder
1/2 tsp dried oregano
sea salt to taste
pepper to taste
3 leaves Boston, bibb or butterhead lettuce
6 leaves Belgian endive

Toss together all ingredients except lettuce and endive. Chill. Place on serving platter atop fan of lettuce and endive leaves.

Yield: 6 servings

NUTRI-NOTE: Using sprouted chickpeas will greatly increase the nutritional value of this salad.

*"Nature feels she owes you good health
and is willing at all times to pay her debt!
but you must at least do your part....
Try to conform with what nature demands
in the form of a sensible diet...."*

Dr. Joseph Franklin Montague

Cole Slaw

1 head cabbage, grated
2 large carrots, peeled and grated
1 T celery seed
1 egg yolk
1 tsp lemon juice
1/4 tsp sea salt
1/4 C honey
1/4 C Dijon mustard
1/4 C extra virgin olive oil
fresh ground pepper to taste

Mix cabbage, carrots and celery seed together in a large bowl. Blend egg yolk, lemon juice, sea salt, and honey in a blender. With motor still running, drizzle a thin, steady stream of olive oil through hole in lid and blend until mayonnaise thickens. Toss all ingredients together very well. Stir in a few shakes of pepper and serve.

Yield: 4 servings

HELPFUL HINT:
If mayo is too thick, thin with a teaspoon of hot water.

"There is a whole category of substances that have a far more intense effect on our patients than drugs. That category is food...."

David Reuben, MD

Date Waldorf Salad with Banana Dressing

1/2 C dates, pitted and chopped
1 apple, chopped
1 stalk celery, diced
1/4 C walnuts, chopped
3 leaves Boston or Romaine lettuce
2 very ripe bananas, mashed
2 T hazelnuts, finely ground
1 tsp honey
2 tsp lemon juice

To make dressing, thoroughly mix bananas, hazelnuts, honey and lemon juice and let stand for 15 minutes. Combine chopped dates, apples, walnuts, and celery with dressing. Serve on lettuce leaves.

Yield: 3 servings

TASTY TIP:
For a nice variation, substitute raisins for dates.

"...Since our bodies are 70 percent water, we should be eating a diet that is approximately 70 percent water content, and that means fruits and vegetables should predominate in our diets."

Harvey Diamond

Dijon Vinaigrette

2 tsp Dijon mustard
1/2 tsp garlic, minced
4 tsp red wine vinegar
1/2 C extra virgin olive oil
1/2 tsp rosemary, ground
1 tsp honey
1 tsp water
dash sea salt
pepper to taste

Place all ingredients into blender and mix at medium speed.

Yield: 1/2 cup

*"Many people just simply are not aware...
that what they eat, or do not eat,
has a profound influence on their health."*

William H. Sebrell, Jr., MD

Eden Spice Dressing

1 avocado
1 red bell pepper
2 scallions, chopped
2 T lemon juice
3/4 C apple juice
1 T liquid aminos
1/2 tsp cumin (to taste)
1/2 tsp cinnamon
1/2 tsp vanilla
dash cayenne (optional)

In a blender, mix all ingredients until smooth and creamy.

Yield: 2 cups

*"Every plant, vegetable, fruit, nut, and seed
in its raw natural state is composed of atoms
and molecules. Within these...reside the vital
elements we know as enzymes...the life principle
in the atoms and molecules of every living cell."*

Norman Walker, DSc, PhD

Hawaiian Beet Salad

1 large beet, tops removed, cut into chunks
1 C chopped fresh pineapple
1/2 C unsweetened shredded coconut
5 leaves Boston lettuce

Shred beet in food processor. Toss with pineapple chunks and coconut. Scoop onto lettuce leaves.

Yield: 5 servings

HELPFUL HINT:
Beets may turn your urine or stool red. You are not bleeding.

"Cultivate the salad habit as if your life depended on it — it does!"

Doris Grant

Hazelnut Dijon Dressing

2 T hazelnut oil
2 T extra virgin olive oil
4 T fresh lemon juice
2 T Dijon mustard
2 tsp maple syrup

In a bowl, whisk together all ingredients. Pour over salad and serve.

Yield: 4-6 servings

*"Three important factors...interfere with
the proper chemicals getting to...
our bloodstream – and these...
are the [depleted] soil, the processing
...of foods...and the cooking of our foods."*

Dr. Bernard Jensen

Hearty Salad

6 leaves romaine lettuce, shredded
1 scallion, chopped
1 ripe avocado, sliced
1/2 zucchini, sliced thinly
1/2 red pepper, cut into 1 inch squares
1/2 C pine nuts

Place greens on salad plates. Arrange remaining vegetables atop greens. Sprinkle with pine nuts. Serve with balsamic vinaigrette dressing.

Yield: 2 servings

"If you want to be vibrantly and vigorously alive, in the best possible shape, you have to eat food that's alive."

Harvey Diamond

Herb Dressing

1/2 tsp ground thyme
1/4 tsp ground marjoram or rosemary
1/4 tsp ground tarragon
1/2 tsp ground basil
1/4 tsp dried oregano
1 tsp dried parsley
1/4 tsp sea salt
1/2 tsp honey
1/4 tsp minced garlic
pinch pepper
1/2 C extra virgin olive oil
3 T apple cider vinegar

Place all ingredients into covered jar. Shake vigorously until well mixed. Allow to stand in refrigerator for at least one hour for flavors to blend.

Yield: 3/4 cup

"Never before have so many members of a mammalian species eaten so much, burned away so little...and accumulated so much surplus fat."

Drs. S. Boyd Eaton and Melvin Konner

Lemon Tamari Dressing

1 C pine nuts, ground to a fine powder
4 T lemon juice
1 T tamari
1 tsp maple syrup
1 tsp sesame oil
2 T water

Place all ingredients in a blender. Puree 2-3 minutes until creamy.

Yield: 1/2 cup

HELPFUL HINT:
For digestibility, soak pine nuts for 6 hours in water to cover. Drain and place directly into blender.

"Food, to sustain life and health and to permit growth, must be organic in form. Inorganic substances...stimulate, but at the same time may also poison insidiously."

Henry Biehler, MD

Orange Tahini Dressing

1 C orange juice
3 T raw sesame tahini
4 dates
1 clove garlic, minced
dash ginger (optional)

Soak dates overnight in water to cover; drain.
Place all ingredients except juice into blender.
Gradually add juice and blend until smooth and
creamy.

Yield: 1 cup

NUTRI-NOTE:
Raw sesame
seeds contain
more calcium
than any other
food on earth.

*"The great Law of Life is replenishment. If we
do not eat, we die. Just as surely, if we do not
eat the kind of food which will nourish the body
constructively, we not only die prematurely
but we suffer along the way."*

Norman Walker, DSc, PhD

Oriental Sprout Salad

4 C mixed Asian greens
2 C mung, aduki, sunflower or other sprouts
1 C red pepper, seeded and sliced thinly
1 C celery, thinly sliced on diagonal
1 C fresh snow pea pods
1 C chopped Chinese cabbage
1/2 C diced scallions
1 C mandarin orange slices
1/2 C slivered almonds

Place bed of mixed Asian greens on salad plates.
Toss together celery, pepper, cabbage, snow
peas and scallions and arrange atop greens.
Combine sprouts and place one-half cup on each
plate. Garnish with almonds and orange slices.
Serve with orange-tahini dressing.

Yield: 6-8 servings

NUTRI-NOTE:
Seeds contain all
the elements
needed for life
and growth.
Sprouting
increases the
nutritional value of
a seed about a
hundredfold.

*"It is not the food in your life but the life
in your food that counts!"*

John H. Tobe

Papaya Seed Vinaigrette

1/2 C fresh papaya seeds
1 C papaya nectar (fruit sweetened)
1/4 C apple cider vinegar
1/4 C Dijon mustard
1/8 C fresh lime juice
2 T shallots, chopped
1/2 tsp sea salt
2 oz. extra virgin olive oil
1 tsp raw honey

Place all ingredients in a food processor and blend until pureed well.

Yield: 2 cups

NUTRI-NOTE:
Papaya seeds are rich in papain, an effective protein-digesting enzyme.

"The foods we eat today and the foods our children eat will determine the diseases we develop tomorrow."

Delia Garcia, MD

Pear and Water Chestnut Salad with Lemon Maple Dressing

1 pear, peeled, cored and chopped
8 oz can water chestnuts, drained and diced
1/2 C Brazil nuts, chopped
12-16 orange segments
8 large Romaine lettuce leaves
1/4 C red cabbage, finely shredded
2 tsp maple syrup
2 T lemon juice

Tear lettuce leaves into bite-sized pieces. Toss with cabbage. Combine lemon juice and syrup in a bowl. Add pears, water chestnuts and Brazil nuts and mix well. Spoon onto lettuce-cabbage bed. Surround with orange segments.

Yield: 2 servings

TASTY TIP:
3/4 C sunchokes, peeled and diced, may be substituted for water chestnuts.

"One-fourth of what we eat keeps us alive;
three-fourths of what we eat
keeps the doctor alive."

Benjamin Franklin

Quinoa Tabouli

1 1/4 C cooked quinoa
1 medium tomato, finely chopped
1 small cucumber, peeled and diced
2/3 C minced scallions (about 4)
1 green pepper, diced
1 C finely chopped parsley
1 tsp dried mint or 1/4 C chopped fresh mint (
1/4 C cold pressed sesame or olive oil
3/8 C lemon juice
1/2 tsp sea salt

Mix together all ingredients and chill.

Yield: 3 cups

TASTY TIP:
One cup
cracked or
sprouted wheat
may be
substituted for
quinoa.

*"If anything is true about nutrition, it is that...
when man first appeared on this earth, there
were present all the cyclical food chains
necessary to nourish man and all the
animals and plant life on the land,
in the waters, and in the air."*

Bernard A. Bellow, MD

Radicchio Salad with Hazelnut Dressing

1/2 C hazelnuts (filberts), chopped
1/2 small head radicchio
1/4 head Romaine lettuce
6 Belgian endive leaves
2 large white mushrooms, sliced
2 T lemon juice
2 T extra virgin olive oil
1 T maple syrup

Clean and shred all leafy vegetables. Toss with mushrooms and set aside. Combine lemon juice, oil, maple syrup and hazelnuts. Toss salad leaves with nut dressing until well coated.

Yield: 2-3 servings

"There are hundreds of thousands of cases of sickness and thousands upon thousands of deaths every year simply because people do not know... how to eat and what to eat."

Dr. William J. Robinson

Rainbow Root Salad

1-2 heads Boston, bibb or butterhead lettuce
1 large parsnip
1 large carrot
1 medium beet

Remove large outer leaves of lettuce. Arrange 4-5 small lettuce leaves around plates, core side in. Shred separately parsnip, carrot and beet. Place shredded vegetables in small mounds in center of lettuce fan. Serve chilled with herb dressing.

Yield: 5-6 servings

"Any food which has been cooked at a temperature higher than 130 degrees F. has been subjected to the death sentence of its enzymes, and is nothing but dead food."

Norman Walker, DSc, PhD

Spinach Salad with Orange Vinaigrette

4 C baby spinach leaves
1 can (11 oz) mandarin oranges, drained
1 C fresh sliced mushrooms
3/4 C walnuts, chopped
1/3 C sliced red onion
1/4 C extra virgin olive oil
1/4 C apple cider vinegar
1/4 C orange juice
1/4 C maple syrup

Arrange spinach, mushrooms, and onions on chilled salad plates. Top with mandarin oranges and chopped walnuts. In a small bowl, stir together remaining four ingredients and pour dressing over salad.

Yield: 4 servings

NUTRI-NOTE: Calcium is abundant in green leafy veggies like spinach.

"When we live on denatured foods...our body reacts with an increase of white blood corpuscles."

Ebba Waerland

Sprouted Sunflower Salad

2 C sunflower sprouts
4 C spring greens
1 C shredded carrots
1 C sliced sunchokes (Jerusalem artichokes)

Toss greens and sunchokes and place on salad plates. Arrange carrots atop greens. Garnish liberally with sunflower sprouts. Serve with Dijon vinaigrette (see above).

Yield: 4 servings

"Today more than 3000 chemicals are deliberately added to our foods. How much do we know about the hazards to human health from these chemicals?"

Senator Abraham Ribicoff

Three Bean Salad

2 C cooked or canned kidney or black beans,
   drained
2 C cooked or canned black-eye peas or white
   beans
2 C chopped cooked green beans
1 small red onion, diced
1 T dried parsley
1/4 C honey
1/4 C apple cider vinegar
1/4 C extra virgin olive oil
1/2 tsp dried basil
1 tsp Dijon mustard

Stir all beans together and set aside. Mix all
remaining ingredients together to make a
marinade. Marinate beans for at least 2 hours.
Chill and serve.

Yield: 6 cups

NUTRI-NOTE:
Beans contain
substantial
amounts of fiber
and protease
inhibitors, which
help keep cancer
in check.

*"I will prevent disease wherever I can,
for prevention is preferable to cure."*

Louis Lasagna, MD

Tropical Salad

2 mangos, peeled and seeded
2 avocados, peeled
1 large papaya, peeled and seeded
4 C mesclun spring greens
4 oz cashews, chopped finely
6 oz papaya seed vinaigrette (see above)

Slice fruits into thin slices. Mix greens with 2 oz vinaigrette. Divide into 4 portions and mound onto salad plates. Surround with sliced fruit, alternating in a swirl pattern. Drizzle remaining vinaigrette over fruit and top with chopped cashews.

Yield: 4 servings

"Almost every medical condition is either caused by or affected in some way by what we eat."

Isadore Rosenfeld, MD

Vegan Caesar Dressing

6 T raw pine nuts, finely ground
2 large cloves garlic, minced
2 T Dijon mustard
2 T lemon juice
1 T tamari
1/2 C water
1 T extra virgin olive oil
1/2 tsp maple syrup
pinch pepper

Blend all ingredients at medium speed until creamy.

Yield: 1 cup

"Nature has given us food...perfect for man's utilization, but we are not content. We mutilate...refine, polish, and separate it into fractions; hold it in...cans or packages for indefinite periods; add chemical preservatives; cook it carelessly; and finally add vitamins and minerals to make it fit for human consumption."

N. Philip Norman, MD

Wild Rice and Peach Salad

1 C wild rice, rinsed well
3 C water
1 1/4 tsp sea salt
2 T extra virgin olive oil
1 T lemon juice
1 clove garlic, minced
3 C chopped fresh peaches
2 scallions, thinly sliced
1/2 tsp dried coriander
8 C mixed spring greens

Bring wild rice, water, and 1 tsp salt to boil. Cover and simmer about 50 minutes, until rice is tender and water is absorbed. Whisk olive oil with lemon juice, garlic, and 1/4 tsp salt. Stir into hot wild rice. Refrigerate, uncovered, until cool. Stir in peaches, scallions, and coriander. Serve on bed of greens.

Yield: 8 servings

TASTY TIP:
For variation, substitute chopped nectarines or mangos for some or all of the peaches.

"The type and quality of [the] food you eat has a profound influence on your health."

Dr. Joseph Mercola

ENTREES & SIDES

Acorn Squash with Quinoa Pilaf

2 large acorn squash
1 C cooked quinoa
2 tsp extra virgin olive oil
1 onion, finely chopped
1/4 lb shitake mushrooms, finely chopped
2 T fresh parsley, finely chopped
1/4 tsp Herbamare seasoning
1 tsp Mrs. Dash seasonings, ground in mill
4 tsp honey

Preheat oven to 350 F. Carefully cut squash in half at equator. Trim ends so squash sits level. Scoop out seeds. Place cut side down in baking pan with 1/4 inch of water and bake for 40 minutes. In a saucepan, saute onion in olive oil for 5 minutes over medium heat. Add mushrooms and saute for 3 more minutes. Add parsley and seasonings and stir into cooked quinoa. Stuff squash with quinoa mixture. Place in baking pan. Pour a thin drizzle of honey around squash tops. Bake for 15 minutes.

Yield: 4 servings

"People who eat raw food never eat too much."

John H. Tobe

Asparagus Hollandaise

1 lb fresh asparagus spears
3 egg yolks
4 tsp lemon juice
1/4 tsp sea salt
dash cayenne pepper
1/4 lb unsalted butter

Trim and carefully wash asparagus. Place over water in steamer basket, cover, and bring to a boil. Reduce heat to medium and steam about 6 minutes or until just tender. Heat butter in double boiler over hot water until just melted. In a blender, combine eggs, lemon juice, salt and pepper. Blend at high speed for 30 seconds. While blender is running, drizzle butter slowly through hole in top. Place asparagus on serving plates and spoon on sauce.

Yield: 3 servings

TASTY TIP:
Asparagus should be tender but not mushy; do not overcook.

"Virtually every disease of aging...results from damage to DNA, which can be prevented by the substances found in fruits and vegetables."

David Heber, MD, PhD

Baked Stuffed Peppers

1 medium onion, finely chopped
2 cloves garlic, minced
1 T extra virgin olive oil
2 celery stalks, finely chopped
4 T fresh parsley, chopped
2 C cooked brown rice
1/2 tsp salt
4 large sweet bell peppers (yellow, red, orange, green)
1/2 C ground pecans
1/4 C raw sunflower seeds

Preheat oven to 350 F. Saute onion and garlic in oil for about 1 minute. Add celery and saute 3 minutes. Mix with remaining ingredients. Cut off stems and about 1/2 inch of pepper tops. Clean out seeds, wash and pat dry. Stuff peppers with sautéed mixture, packing tightly. Replace pepper tops. Place in casserole dish with 1/8 inch of water. Heat thoroughly 15-18 minutes.

Yield: 4 servings

*"The over-eating of refined foods
is the only form of suicide
tolerated by our customs."*

Dr. Clive McCay

Carrot Nut Loaf

1 C grated carrots
1 C walnuts, finely chopped
1/4 C raw sunflower seeds
1 C cooked quinoa
1 small onion, diced finely
2 eggs, well beaten
1/2 stalk celery, finely chopped
pinch sea salt
dash pepper
1/8 tsp garlic powder
3/4 C tomato paste
1 1/2 T honey
3/8 tsp dried basil
1/4 tsp dried oregano

Preheat oven to 325 F. Combine tomato paste, honey, basil and oregano and set aside. Mix together remaining ingredients. Spoon into oiled 1 qt loaf pan. Bake at 325 F for 25 minutes. Remove from oven and spread with 1/4 inch thick layer of tomato paste. Bake another 15 minutes. Allow to cool slightly before cutting into 6 equal slices.

Yield: 6 servings

HELPFUL HINT: Use sharp knife, non-serrated, to loosen loaf from pan sides, and cut slices with smooth motion.

"Nothing offends patients more than to be asked to change their habits of life."

Alexander Bryce, MD

Carrot Zucchini Squares

3 eggs, separated
1/4 C honey
1/2 C grated carrots, tightly packed
1/2 C grated zucchini, tightly packed
1/4 C grated and peeled apple
1/4 tsp vanilla extract
1/2 tsp cinnamon (optional)
1/4 C millet flour

Preheat oven to 375 F. In a large mixing bowl, beat the yolks with honey and vanilla. Add carrots, zucchini, apple, cinnamon and flour. Blend well. In another bowl, beat egg whites at high speed until stiff. Gently fold into carrot mixture. Turn into buttered 8 by 8 inch baking pan. Bake for 25 minutes or until puffed and set. Cut into squares and serve warm.

Yield: 9 servings

"Eat with moderation what agrees with your constitution. Nothing is good for the body but what we can digest."

Voltaire

Cashew-Millet Casserole

1 tsp sea salt
2 C cooked millet
2 1/2 T olive oil
1 medium onion, chopped
1 C raw unsalted cashew nuts, ground
3 eggs, beaten
1/4 C chopped parsley
1/2 4-oz jar sliced sweet red pimientos, drained
1/3 C water
1/8 tsp ground rosemary

Preheat oven to 325 F. Heat oil in skillet and saute onion until golden. Combine with cooked millet and ground cashews in a mixing bowl. Add eggs, parsley, and pimento. Stir in water, herbs and salt. Place into oiled 1 1/2 qt casserole and bake uncovered for 50 minutes or until golden brown with firm center. Let cool slightly. Loosen from edges with knife. Cut into wedges or squares.

Yield: 6-8 servings

"By stripping cereals of their outer coats and refining sugar until it is whiter than the whitest snow, we have made a good start on the road to the ruination of human health."

Professors SM Furnas and CC Furnas

Cauliflower and Carrots in Sesame Paste

1 small cauliflower, cut into florets
2 carrots, thinly sliced
1 tsp extra virgin olive oil
1 tsp Dijon mustard
1/2 C raw sesame tahini
1/2 tsp sea salt
1 T lemon juice
1 T honey
3/4 C water

Steam cauliflower and carrots in steamer basket for about 5 minutes. While steaming, combine water, tahini, salt, lemon juice and mustard together in a small bowl. Heat skillet over medium heat. Add oil. Place vegetables in skillet, and cook 1-2 minutes, stirring frequently. Add tahini mixture. Cover and simmer 10 minutes or until vegetables are tender.

Yield: 5-6 servings

HELPFUL HINT:
Do not overcook.

"Rules for healthful eating:
(1) Eat only those foods that spoil or rot or decay, but eat them before they do, and
(2) First eat what you need,
then what you like."

Dr. E. V. McCollum

Chicken Cacciatore

1 large hen, 4-5 lb, skinned and cut into serving
   pieces
3 T extra virgin olive oil
1 large onion, chopped
3 cloves garlic, minced
1 rib celery, chopped
1 C fresh sliced mushrooms
1 jar (25 oz) tomato sauce
pinch sea salt
pinch pepper
1/2 tsp oregano
1/2 C red wine

Heat oil in skillet and saute the chicken until
brown.   Add onion and garlic and saute until they
brown. Add celery, mushrooms, tomato sauce,
and seasonings. Cook slowly for about 1 hour.
5 minutes before serving, add wine.

Yield: 4-5 servings

*"The foods we eat interact intimately with
our genes, and can increase or decrease
our risk of chronic disease."*

David Heber, MD, PhD

Fish Kabobs

1 lb swordfish steaks, cut into 1 1/2 inch chunks
1 onion, cut into 1 1/2 inch wedges
1 green pepper, cut into 1 1/2 inch pieces
1 C fresh pineapple chunks
2 fresh peaches
2 tsp apple cider vinegar
1 T honey

Blend together peaches, vinegar and honey. Marinate fish, onion and peppers in peach mixture for 1 hour. Thread items onto skewers, alternating fish, onion, pepper, and pineapple. Grill or broil for about 15 minutes, turning frequently.

Yield: 3-4 servings

NUTRI-NOTE
Do not overcook. Charring causes formation of carcinogenic compounds.

"Improper eating, living and thinking habits are the prime cause of degeneration."

Sir James Mackenzie, MD

Flounder Florentine

1/4 C onion, finely chopped
1 T extra virgin olive oil
1/2 lb fresh baby spinach leaves, washed
1/3 C cooked brown rice
1/4 C chopped fresh mushrooms
1 tsp lemon juice
4 flounder fillets (about 3/4 lb), rinsed and patted
   dry

Preheat oven to 350 F. In a large skillet, saute
onion and mushrooms in oil until golden. Add
spinach and saute just enough to wilt the spinach
(about 3 minutes). Stir in rice and lemon juice.
Place about 1/4 C of the mixture on each fish
fillet. Roll and secure with a toothpick. Arrange
in oiled, shallow baking dish (10 by 6 by 2 inches)
and bake for 20 minutes.

Yield: 2 servings

TASTY TIP:
Serve with warm
tomato sauce if
desired.

*"Your body is made out of foods and can be
no better than the foods you eat."*

R.G. Jackson, MD

Glazed Carrots and Parsnips

2 C parsnips, thinly sliced into 1/8 inch pennies
2 C fresh carrots, thinly sliced
3 T honey
1 tsp salt
1 tsp grated orange peel
2 tsp butter
dash cinnamon

Steam carrots and parsnips over water for 8 minutes or until tender. Cook honey, salt, orange peel and butter in a skillet until bubbly, stirring occasionally. Add vegetables and cook over low heat for about 2 minutes or until glazed. Sprinkle with dash of cinnamon.

Yield: 5 servings

NUTRI-NOTE:
Parsnips are low in calories, high in complex carbohydrates and insoluble fiber, and a useful source of vitamin C and folate.

"Health depends upon nutrition more than on any other single factor in hygiene."

William H. Sebrell, Jr., MD

Lentil Loaf with Mushroom Gravy

2 1/2 C cooked brown lentils
1/4 medium onion, diced
1 tsp extra virgin olive oil
1/2 C ground flaxseeds
1 C cooked brown rice
1 egg, beaten
1/2 C chopped walnuts
1/4 tsp ground thyme
1/8 tsp oregano
1 tsp Mrs. Dash blend, ground
1/2 T apple cider vinegar
1 tsp Sucanat
sea salt to taste

Preheat oven to 350 F. Saute onion in olive oil until soft. Mix all ingredients together in a bowl. Place in large oiled loaf pan. Cover and bake 40 minutes.

Yield: 6-8 servings

Mushroom Gravy

1 C raw cashews, finely ground
8 oz can sliced mushrooms, with liquid
1/2 tsp Herbamare
2 T vegetable broth
2 T water
dash pepper

Puree all ingredients together in blender. Heat slowly, stirring frequently, until warm. Spoon over loaf slices.

Pasta Primavera

10 oz package whole grain pasta
2 cloves garlic, minced
1 small red onion, sliced
12 shitake or button mushrooms, sliced
1 T fresh basil, minced
1 T fresh parsley, minced
1 T fresh oregano, minced
1 zucchini, cut into thin strips
2 red peppers, cut into thin strips
2 C small broccoli florets
3 T extra virgin olive oil
2 C tomato pasta sauce

Over medium heat, saute garlic and onion 2
minutes in 4 T water, stirring occasionally. Add
broccoli and cook one minute. Add red pepper,
zucchini and mushrooms and cook for 5 minutes
more. Add herbs and olive oil, cover, and remove
from heat. Boil pasta according to directions.
Drain and combine with vegetables. Toss well
with warmed tomato sauce.

Yield: 5 servings

HELPFUL HINT:
1 1/2 teaspoons
of dried herbs
may be
substituted for
each fresh herb.

*"... fine milling removes 75% of the minerals.
Super-refinement has probably been as
successful in promoting American ill-health...
as the most virulent disease germs."*

Professors SM Furnas and CC Furnas

Pineapple Chicken

8 boneless breasts of chicken, skinned
1/3 C honey
4 C pineapple chunks
1/4 C lemon juice
1/4 tsp sea salt
1/4 tsp pepper
1/4 tsp oregano
1/4 tsp minced garlic
1 T extra virgin olive oil

Preheat oven to 400 degrees F. Place chicken
breasts in glass baking dish. Place pineapple into
food processor and process until crushed. Mix
pineapple with all remaining ingredients. Pour
over chicken. Bake one hour, turning at least
once.

Yield: 6-8 servings

HELPFUL HINT:
If need be,
substitute 1 large
can crushed
pineapple –
it's faster.

*"If the doctors of today do not become the
nutritionists of tomorrow, then the nutritionists
of today will become the doctors of tomorrow."*

Rockefeller Institute of Medical Research

Portobello Mushroom Burgers

4 C walnuts
1 lb carrots, scrubbed and cut in pieces
1 medium onion, chopped
5 cloves garlic, minced
1 T honey
1 T extra virgin olive oil
2 T flaxseeds, finely ground
1 1/2 T poultry seasoning or Mrs. Dash seasoning
sea salt to taste
2 large, ripe tomatoes, sliced
1 large red onion, sliced
9 portobello mushroom caps, washed and patted
   dry
18 leaves fresh spinach

Grind walnuts in food processor until coarsely chopped. Set aside. Process carrots until finely ground. Add chopped onion, garlic, honey, oil, flaxseeds and seasonings and process until well blended. Add walnuts to carrot mixture and process a few seconds. Form into 9 patties. Place mushroom caps upside down on platter. Place 2 spinach leaves over each mushroom. Place patties atop spinach, tomato slices atop burgers, and onion slices atop tomatoes. Secure the sandwich with a toothpick. Warm in oven at low temperature for a few minutes before serving.

Yield: 9 servings

"I saw a few die of hunger –
of eating, a hundred thousand."

Benjamin Franklin

Quinoa with Peppers

1 C quinoa
2 C water
1 C red bell peppers, thinly sliced in julienne
    strips
1 C green bell peppers, julienned
1 C yellow peppers, julienned
4 large mushrooms, sliced thinly
1 large onion, chopped
1 C cooked kidney beans
3 T extra virgin olive oil
pinch sea salt (optional)

Bring water to a boil. Add quinoa, cover, and
simmer 20 minutes or until all water has been
absorbed. While quinoa is cooking, stir fry
peppers, mushrooms and onions over medium
heat for 10 minutes, stirring occasionally. Warm
kidney beans in a few drops of water, stirring
frequently, and drain. Place 1 C quinoa in center
of each plate. Surround with ring of pepper
mixture and top with 1/2 C kidney beans.

Yield: 2 servings

NUTRI-NOTE:
Quinoa is a high-
protein grain rich
in all 8 essential
amino acids.

*"In all considerations of health or illness,
the manner and the matter of food
rank so much higher than all others...."*

William Howard Hay, MD

Rice Pilaf

1 T extra virgin olive oil
1 medium onion, chopped
2 C uncooked basmati rice
3 1/2 C water
1 T unsalted butter
1/2 C raisins
1/2 C shelled whole pistachio nuts
1/2 tsp sea salt
2 T Chinese five spice

In a large saucepan, sauté onion in olive oil over medium heat until translucent. Add water, rice, and salt and bring to a boil. Add butter, lower heat, and simmer 20 minutes. Add raisins, pistachio nuts, and spices and simmer 10 minutes more.

Yield: 5 servings

TASTY TIP:
Chinese five spice is a blend of fennel, anise, licorice, ginger, cinnamon and/or cloves. If desired, experiment with any combination of these.

"Cancerous cells will only grow in a suitable soil, and that soil is provided by the prolonged action of the toxins in the tissues."

Sir William Arbuthnot Lane, MD

Salmon Leek Pie

4 large leeks
2 T unsalted butter or olive oil
4 lbs. wild Alaskan salmon fillets, skinned
1 T chopped dill (optional)
1 tsp lemon zest
1 1/2 tsp sea salt
1/4 tsp black pepper
1 package phyllo sheets

Preheat oven to 400 F. Cut white and green parts of leeks crosswise into 1/2 inch wide slices. Wash well in cold water, rinse and dry. In a large skillet, cook leeks in butter over moderate heat about 12 minutes, stirring frequently. Remove from pan and cool. Cut salmon into 3/4 inch pieces. In a bowl, toss salmon, leeks, dill, zest, salt and pepper until well combined.

Grease a 9 by 12 inch baking sheet. Place phyllo sheet on pan and brush with olive oil. Repeat until half of the sheets have been used. Spread fish filling over top layer of phyllo. Continue to add phyllo layers until completed. Cut into serving size pieces with a sharp knife. Bake pie 30-40 minutes until golden brown.

Yield: 12-16 servings

NUTRI-NOTE:
Wild Alaskan salmon is superior to farm raised salmon. The former has healthy omega-3 fats; the latter is high in saturated fats and is often treated with carcinogenic dyes.

Sauteed Arugula

6 oz arugula leaves
2 large cloves garlic, minced
2 T extra virgin olive oil
dash sea salt

Wash greens well. Cook garlic in olive oil for
about 15 seconds. Add arugula and cook for
about 30 seconds more.

Yield: 2 servings

NUTRI-NOTE:
This recipe may
be tried with any
type of bitter
greens, all
valuable for
cleansing the
liver.

*"Scientists say that in nearly every household
the food is prepared...in a way that removes
70 to 80 percent of its essential minerals
and vitamins."*

Bruce Bliven

Snow Peas and Sprouts with Rice

4 C cooked medium grain brown rice
1/4 tsp sea salt
4 C snow peas
4 C mung bean sprouts
4 T extra virgin olive oil
2 large cloves garlic, minced
1 medium onion, chopped
1 1/2 C fresh mushrooms, sliced

Over medium heat, saute onion and mushrooms in 2 T olive oil for 2 minutes or until golden. Stir into rice. Add salt and mix well. Saute garlic in 2 T olive oil for 30 seconds, stirring frequently. Add snow peas and continue to stir for 1 minute more. Add mung sprouts and saute for an additional 45 seconds. Serve over brown rice mixture.

Yield: 4 large servings

"All the chemicals used in the body — except for the oxygen we breathe and the water we drink – are taken in through food.... All disease could be prevented and...cured through proper nutrition."

Tom Douglas Spies, MD

Stir-Fried Kale

3/4 lb dinosaur kale (1-2 bunches)
2 T extra virgin olive oil
1 onion, chopped
2 cloves garlic, minced
1/4 C walnuts, chopped
1/4 C flaxseeds, ground

Wash kale well and pat dry. Pull kale leaves away from thick stems and shred into 2-3 inch pieces. Heat oil over medium heat in large frying pan. Add onions and garlic and cook until soft and golden. Stir in kale and cook until wilted, turning leaves frequently. Combine ground flax and walnuts and sprinkle atop kale just before serving.

Yield: 4 servings

NUTRI-NOTE:
Dark green veggies like kale are loaded with calcium.

"Malnutrition leads to immunosuppression as well as do surgery, radiation therapy and chemotherapy....There is increasing clinical evidence that re-establishment of cellular immunity by nutritional means...plays an important role in decreasing morbidity and mortality."

Maurice Shils, MD, ScD

Sweet Potato Casserole

10 large sweet potatoes, scrubbed and sliced
1 C honey
2 tsp cinnamon
1/2 tsp salt
4 cans (11 oz) mandarin orange segments,
    drained
1 tsp vanilla

Preheat oven to 325 F. Grate potatoes in processor. In a large mixing bowl, combine potatoes, honey, salt, cinnamon and vanilla. Stir well. Fold in mandarin oranges. Place in 9 by 12 by 2 inch casserole pan. Bake 1 hour, uncovered.

Yield: 8-10 servings

HELPFUL HINT:
Four 29-ounce cans of vacuum packed sweet potatoes can be substituted if necessary. Oven time will greatly decrease: Heat through and serve.

"We send our children to the best schools we can afford, and try to equip them with moral values that will last a lifetime, but we give them food habits that, when they grow up, will cut short two lives out of every three."

Neal Barnard, MD

Thai Curry Chicken

4 boneless skinless chicken breasts, cut into
   bite-sized pieces
1 can light coconut milk
2 T curry
2 T honey
1 onion or 2 scallions, sliced
basil to taste

Place all ingredients in wok and cook, covered,
over high heat for 25 minutes. Stir occasionally.
Serve over basmati rice.

Yield: 4 servings

"Doctors are looking for a cure while, truly,
our bodies are just suffering
from a hidden hunger."

Dr. Bernard Jensen

Turkey Piccata with Artichokes and Peppers

2 lbs turkey breast, sliced into 1 by 2 inch strips
2 cans artichoke hearts in water, drained and
    halved
1/2 C lemon juice
1 C fresh sliced mushrooms
2 large fresh red peppers, julienned
2 tsp garlic powder
2 tsp oregano
1/2 tsp pepper
1/2 tsp salt
1/4 C extra virgin olive oil
1 lemon, thinly sliced

Saute turkey slices in olive oil over medium heat.
Set aside. Saute peppers and mushrooms in
remaining oil until soft. Add artichokes, turkey,
lemon juice and spices and cook covered over
low heat about 10 minutes. Garnish with lemon
slices and serve.

Yield: 6 servings

*"Trying to beat cancer while eating a diet
that constantly raises blood glucose is like
trying to put out a forest fire while somebody
...is throwing gasoline on the trees."*

Patrick Quillin, PhD

Vegetable Puffs

2 medium onions, chopped
1 lb. fresh mushrooms, coarsely chopped
4 T extra virgin olive oil
40 oz frozen chopped spinach, defrosted and drained
8 carrots, peeled and grated
8 eggs, lightly beaten
1 tsp salt
1/2 tsp black pepper
1 C matzo meal

Preheat oven to 350 F. Grease three 12-cup muffin tins. Saute onions and mushrooms in skillet and set aside. Add spinach, carrots, onions, mushrooms, salt, pepper and matzoh meal to beaten eggs. Mix thoroughly. Put mixture in muffin tins and bake for 45 minutes. Release puffs from muffin tins with a narrow spatula. Serve warm.

Yield: 36 puffs

HELPFUL HINT:
Do not overbake.

"The same father who would run in front of a speeding car to push a child out of danger nods approvingly as his daughters or sons learn eating habits that will later take their lives."

Neal Barnard, MD

Wild Rice Supreme

2 C wild rice
4 C water
1 1/2 tsp sea salt
2 C fresh mushrooms, sliced
1/3 C unsalted butter
1 C raw cashews
2 tsp chopped parsley

Rinse rice thoroughly in a sieve under running water for 2 minutes. Place in large saucepan with water. Bring to a boil. Turn heat down, add salt and cook, covered, until nearly all water has been absorbed and rice is tender, about 1 hour. Sautee mushrooms in butter for about 5 minutes, stirring frequently. Process cashews in a coffee mill until finely ground. Add nuts, mushrooms and parsley to rice, toss well and simmer another 3 minutes.

Yield: 8-10 servings

HELPFUL HINT: Two 8 oz. cans of sliced mushrooms may be substituted. Drain and add to rice without sauteeing.

"Food alone cures most diseases."

Hu-Sei-Hui

SWEETS & TREATS

Almond Macaroons

2 cups raw, unblanched almonds
3/4 C honey
2 egg whites
1 1/2 tsp pure vanilla extract
2/3 C unsweetened, shredded coconut

Preheat oven to 425 F. Pulverize almonds and coconut in processor. Gradually blend honey into ground almonds until mixture forms a dense ball. In electric mixing bowl, beat egg whites at high speed until stiff peaks form. Slowly beat in the almond mixture until thoroughly combined. Add vanilla extract. Using a teaspoon, shape mixture into 1 1/2 inch balls and arrange two inches apart on an oiled cookie sheet. Bake for 7 minutes or until golden. Remove cookies from pan and place on a wire rack to cool.

Yield: About 3 dozen cookies

NUTRI-NOTE:
Just one ounce of raw almonds provides 35 % of the RDA of vitamin E, 3 grams of fiber, and 75 mg of calcium.

"Over 40% of cancer patients actually die from malnutrition, not from the cancer."

Patrick Quillin, PhD

Apple Cobbler

Crust:

3/4 C raw almonds
3/4 C pecans
1 1/2 C dates, pitted
1/4 C flaxseeds, ground
1/4 tsp ground cinnamon

Soak almonds in water to cover for 12 hours. Rinse and drain. Grind flaxseeds in coffee mill. Process almonds, pecans, and dates until well ground. Add flax and cinnamon and process again to incorporate into nut mixture. Set aside half of crust to use as topping. Press remaining crust into bottom of 9 by 6 inch pan.

Filling:

3 C apples, peeled, cored and chopped
1 T flaxseeds, ground
2 T psyllium husks
2/3 C fresh apple juice
1 1/2 tsp lemon juice
pinch of allspice
pinch of cinnamon

Mix together psyllium, flaxseeds, apple juice and lemon juice. Combine with apples. Add spices. Place apple mixture onto crust and top with leftover crust mixture. Serve cold or warmed.

Yield: 8 fiber-filled servings

Baked Pears

2 fresh, ripe bartlett pears, cored, peeled, and
    halved
2 T water
1 T maple syrup
1/2 tsp vanilla extract
2 tsp flaxseeds, finely ground
4 pecan halves, finely ground

Preheat oven to 350 F. Place 2 T water into glass
baking dish. Place pears in dish, cored side
down. Mix syrup and vanilla extract. Drizzle over
pears. Bake 10 minutes. Stir together flax and
pecans. Sprinkle over pears. Serve warm.

Yield: 2-4 servings

*"The traditional four food groups and the
eating patterns they prescribed have killed
more people than any other factor in America."*

Neal Barnard, MD

Banana Apple Pudding

2 medium apples, grated
16 raw almonds, ground
2 ripe bananas
2 tsp. grated unsweetened coconut

Mash all but half of one banana. Combine mashed banana with apples and nuts. Place into small dessert bowls. Sprinkle with grated coconut. Decorate with slices of remaining half banana. Chill.

Yield: 2-3 servings

"Our brilliant researchers have spent 30 years and $45 billion of your tax dollars wrestling with the complex issue of curing cancer. Yet Nature has been solving the dilemma for thousands of years."

Patrick Quillin, PhD

Banana Cream Pie

Crust

2 C pecans
8 pitted dates
1/2 tsp vanilla
dash cinnamon
1 T water

In a food processor, process the pecans until uniformly fine. Add dates and process until they are fully blended and the mixture is sticky. Add vanilla, cinnamon, and enough water to hold the crust together. Press into an 8 or 9 inch pie pan.

Filling

6 ripe bananas, frozen
1 C unsweetened coconut
1/2 C dates, pitted and chopped
1 tsp vanilla

Soak dates for 15 minutes in enough water to cover them. Drain well. Process together coconut, dates, and vanilla and set aside. Push frozen bananas through a Champion juicer, using the blank screen, and into a chilled bowl. Quickly and gently stir in coconut-date mixture. Pour mixture into crust, smoothing the top with the back of a spoon. Place the pie immediately into freezer and keep frozen for at least four hours.

Yield: 1 pie

HELPFUL HINT:
Remove pie from freezer 15 minutes before serving so it softens for easy slicing.

Banana Ice Cream Sundae

4 ripe bananas, peeled, wrapped in foil, and
   frozen
1/2 C raspberries
1/4 C walnuts, chopped
1/4 C maple syrup

Puree raspberries in blender with maple syrup.
Set aside. Process bananas through Champion
juicer, using solid plate. Quickly place cream into
2 small bowls. Drizzle raspberry sauce over ice
cream. Top with walnuts.

Yield: 2 servings

HELPFUL HINT:
Out of season,
frozen
raspberries may
be used.

*"I sincerely believe that many doctors would
close their offices and go out of business, if
people had the sense of knowing how to eat."*

Dr. R. A. Riggs

Banana Nut Cookies

1 C walnuts
1 C pecans
1 C grated unsweetened coconut
4 ripe bananas, sliced
1/4 C pitted dates
3/4 tsp cinnamon

Preheat oven to 375 F. Place nuts and coconut in a food processor with the S blade and grind to a coarse meal. Add dates and cinnamon. Process bananas into date-nut mixture until it forms a cookie dough. Measure cookies by tablespoons and spoon onto lightly oiled cookie sheet. Bake for 14-15 minutes.

Yield: 2 dozen cookies

TASTY TIP:
Do not overbake. For Banana Pudding, follow recipe exactly as above, omitting the cookie sheet and oven. Spoon into small dessert bowls. Chill. Yield: 2 1/4 cups

"To cure the patient, we must find the cause and change the diet."

Dr. Bernard Jensen

Banana Whip

2 ripe bananas
1 tsp lemon juice
2 oz unsweetened pear juice
1 tsp vanilla
1 T honey
2 T flaxseeds, finely ground
12 Brazil nuts, finely ground
dash cinnamon

Combine ingredients in a blender on the whip setting. Place into dessert bowls. Decorate with a sprinkle of cinnamon. Serve chilled.

Yield: 2 servings

NUTRI-NOTE:
Brazil nuts are rich in selenium, an anti-oxidant mineral important for cancer protection.

"The cause of cancer [lies] in the deficiency of life in the atoms of the food we eat."

Norman Walker, DSc, PhD

Carob Brownies

1 C unsweetened carob powder, sifted
1 C walnut oil
3/4 C honey
4 eggs
1 1/4 C almonds,finely ground in processor or mill
1 C walnuts, chopped
2 tsp vanilla extract

Preheat oven to 325 F. Oil a 9 by 9 by 2 inch pan.
In a small bowl, combine carob powder, oil, vanilla
and honey. In a large mixing bowl, beat eggs until
light. Beat in carob mixture. Stir in almond flour
and mix well. Add chopped nuts. Spread batter
evenly in the prepared pan. Bake for about 30
minutes or just until surface is firm to the touch.
Remove from oven and cool at least 20 minutes
before cutting into squares.

Yield: 16 brownies

HELPFUL HINT:
Do not overbake.
Brownies should
be moist.

*"Miracle anti-cancer agents are waiting
patiently at your nearby grocery store
and health food store."*

Patrick Quillin, PhD

Carob Pudding

1/2 C carob powder
1/4 C medjool dates, pitted
3 large ripe bananas, partially frozen
1 C pine nuts, chilled
1/2 tsp vanilla
1/2 tsp maple syrup
1/2 C chopped walnuts
4 strawberries, sliced

Process all ingredients in processor with an S blade until smooth, adding just enough water to produce a creamy consistency without thinning pudding. Pour into small serving bowls. Sprinkle with chopped walnuts and garnish each with a sliced strawberry fan.

Yield: 4 filling servings

"In America there is such an abundance of food that people are literally eating themselves to death."

Gabriel Cousens, MD

Carob Truffles

1/4 C flaxseeds, ground
1/4 C unsweetened carob powder, sifted
1/3 C walnuts, finely chopped
1/3 C raw almond butter
1/3 C honey
1 tsp vanilla extract
small bowl of unsweetened shredded coconut

Process all ingredients until mixture forms a dense ball. Remove from processor and roll small portions between palms of hands to form one inch balls. Roll in coconut to coat. Place on serving platter and refrigerate.

Yield: Approximately 18 truffles

TASTY TIP:
To make carob fudge, process in an additional 1/4C honey, press into 9 by 9 square pan, and refrigerate. Omit coconut.

"Just as the quality of fuel influences the performance and longevity of an internal combustion engine, so the quality of food we eat must influence the life and health of the body."

Andrew Weil, MD

Carrot Chiffon Cake

1/2 C grated carrots
3/8 C flaked coconut
1/2 tsp vanilla extract
3 eggs, separated
1/2 C raw cashew nuts, finely ground
3/8 C honey
1 tsp arrowroot

In a large bowl, mix carrots, coconut, honey and vanilla. In a separate bowl, beat egg yolks until creamy. Fold yolks into the carrot-coconut mixture and place in freezer 15-20 minutes. Stir in ground cashews. Preheat oven to 400 F. In another bowl, beat egg whites at high speed until stiff. Mix in arrowroot and beat again. Fold egg white mixture into carrot-coconut mixture. Pour into 9-inch pan. Bake at 400 F for 10 minutes, then reduce to 350 F and bake 20 minutes or until cake begins to leave sides of pan. Cool on a wire rack before cutting into squares.

Yield: 9 servings

*"Healthy food and delicious food
are not mutually exclusive."*

Andrew Weil, MD

Cashew Fudge

1 C raw cashews
1/2 C pitted dates
1/2 C raisins
1 heaping T carob powder (optional)
1/2 C fresh pineapple juice
3/8 C ground flaxseeds
1/2 C raw walnuts, coarsely chopped
1 tsp vanilla extract
1 tsp maple syrup

Soak cashews in water to cover for about 8 hours. Drain cashews and place in processor with dates, raisins, carob, and pineapple juice. Process to thick paste. Stir in flaxseed meal and walnuts. Press into ungreased brownie pan (about 1 by 7 by 9 inches) and freeze for 2 hours. Cut into 12 equal rectangular pieces and store in the freezer. Remove from freezer 10 minutes before serving.

Yield: 12 pieces

TASTY TIP:
Omit carob for a delightful vanilla-flavored fudge.

*"Improper foods cause disease;
proper foods cure disease."*

Henry Biehler, MD

Coconut Chews

1 1/2 C raw almonds
1 1/2 C raw cashews
1 T flaxseeds, finely ground
3/4 C honey
1 T vanilla extract
3/4 tsp. sea salt
1 1/2 C unsweetened coconut

Place almonds and cashews in food processor
and pulse until finely chopped but not pulverized.
Add flax, honey, vanilla, coconut and salt and
pulse a few times more. Press firmly into 9 by 5
by 1 inch brownie pan and refrigerate several
hours. Cut into small squares and store in airtight
container in refrigerator.

Yield: About 24 pieces

NUTRI-NOTE:
Flaxseeds are an
excellent source
of omega-3
immune-boosting
fats, and of anti-
cancer chemicals
called lignans.

"...Live foods...with their available enzymes,
anti-oxidants, and phytochemicals,
can be the key to slowing down, and
[even] reversing, premature aging...
heart disease, cancer, and arthritis."

Gary Null, PhD

Coconut Pistachio Pudding

2 1/2 C cooked basmati rice
2 1/2 C unsweetened coconut milk
1/2 C Sucanat natural sweetener
1/2 C raw, unsalted pistachios, coarsely chopped
1 1/2 tsp vanilla extract

Place the rice, coconut milk and Sucanat in a medium-sized saucepan and simmer over low heat for 15 minutes, stirring occasionally, until thick and creamy. Remove from heat and stir in pistachios and vanilla. Let cool to room temperature before serving, or cover and refrigerate to serve chilled.

Yield: 4 servings

NUTRI-NOTE: Sucanat crystals, minimally processed from evaporated cane juice, are rich in vitamins and minerals naturally found in the sugar cane plant.

"We mill our flour and purify our sugar to the point where no self-respecting bug can live on it ....We throw most of the known vitamins to the hogs...and we eat the junk ourselves."

Dr. Wilfred N. Sisk

Fresh Applesauce

2 medium apples, peeled, cored and chopped
1 tsp honey
1/4 C apple juice
1/2 tsp cinnamon
1/2 tsp lemon juice

Process all ingredients together using S blade of processor until sauce is smooth or until desired consistency is reached. Garnish with a dash of cinnamon.

Yield: 1 cup

"Each one of the substances
of a man's diet acts upon his body
and changes it in some way,
and upon these changes
his whole life depends."

Hippocrates

Halvah

1 1/2 C almonds
1/2 C raw tahini
3 T honey
1 tsp vanilla

In a food processor, process almonds until finely ground. Add the tahini, honey and vanilla and process thoroughly. Press onto a plate until it is 1/2 inch thick. Chill in refrigerator for 1 hour or more. Cut into one inch square pieces.

Yield: Approximately 3 dozen pieces

TASTY TIP:
For variation, prepare recipe with 1 tsp lemon juice and top with 1/4 C chopped walnuts, or stir in 2 T well-ground flaxseeds.

"Whatsoever is the father of disease, poor diet is the mother."

Chinese proverb

Lemon Pudding

1 C raw cashews
6 dates, pitted
juice of 3 lemons
2 T maple syrup
2 tsp shredded, unsweetened coconut
1/4 C water

Soak dates in 1/4 C water and cashews in 1 C water for 8-12 hours. Remove dates and set water aside. Rinse, drain and towel dry cashews. In a food processor, combine cashews, dates, maple syrup, and lemon juice and blend until smooth, adding 1/4 C date soak water a few drops at a time. Pour into small dessert bowls. Top with sprinkling of coconut and chill.

Yield: 1 1/2 cups

NUTRI-NOTE:
Soaking the nuts greatly improves their digestibility.

"We must see cancer...as a mandate to make immediate and drastic changes in how we nourish our body."

Mauris Emeka

Maple Walnut Torte

Crust

2 C raw walnuts
8 pitted dates
1/4 tsp vanilla
2 tsp water

In a food processor use the S blade to process the walnuts until uniformly fine. Add dates, vanilla and water and process until the mixture is sticky. Press into a 9-inch pie pan to form crust.

Topping

1 1/2 C raw walnuts
1/2 C pitted dates
1/2 C fresh coconut milk (or canned, sulfite-free)
2 T flaxseeds, finely ground
1 T maple syrup

Process 1 C walnuts, dates and flaxseeds in food processor until smooth. Add coconut milk and maple syrup and process until creamy. Spread onto crust. Garnish with 1/2 C chopped walnuts.

Yield: 10 small but very filling servings

TASTY TIP:
For an interesting variation, try substituting pecans for walnuts and honey for maple syrup.

"Eat wisely, age slowly."

John H. Tobe

Nectarine Sauce with Flaxseeds

3 ripe nectarines, pitted
2 T lemon juice
1/2 T honey
2 T water
dash cinnamon
dash nutmeg
4 T flaxseeds, finely ground

Place all ingredients except flax into food processor, and process with S blade until well blended. Pour into small serving bowls, stir in flax, and serve.

Yield: 2 servings

NUTRI-NOTE: Nectarines are a good source of beta-carotene and protective against epithelial cell cancers of the skin, lungs and throat.

"In parts of the world where the diet consists mostly of fresh fruits and vegetables and whole grains...the risk of cancer is much lower."

David Heber, MD, PhD

Oatmeal Tahini Cookies

5 T tahini
1 1/2 C cut oat groats, coarsely ground
3/4 C honey
1/4 tsp vanilla
1/4 C raisins
1/4 C walnuts
pinch salt
1/2 tsp cinnamon

Preheat oven to 350 F. Put contents of entire jar of tahini in food processor and homogenize. Then place in storage container and measure out 5 T. Put all ingredients into large mixing bowl and stir together. Mixture will be thick. Drop by teaspoonfuls onto oiled baking sheet. Bake 10 minutes.

Yield: About 3 dozen cookies

HELPFUL HINT:
To avoid crumbling cookies when removing from pan, cover cookie sheet in foil, shiny side up, before dropping dough. After baking, place entire pan in freezer for 5-10 minutes. Peel foil backing off cookies.

"Are not our bodies...merely a composite of what we eat and drink daily, yearly, as a life habit?"

William Howard Hay, MD

Pumpkin Pie

2 9-inch, frozen unbaked all natural, whole wheat
    pieshells
1 tsp salt
1 tsp ginger, allspice, or pumpkin pie spices
2 tsp cinnamon
29 oz can pumpkin puree
3/8 C organic apple juice
4 eggs, beaten
1 C honey
2 tsp pure vanilla
1/4 tsp ground cloves (omit if using allspice)
12-16 pecan halves

Preheat oven to 350 F. Place pumpkin puree in a
large mixing bowl. Add eggs, apple juice, honey,
vanilla, and remaining seasonings. Divide evenly
between two pie shells, and bake 30 minutes or
until filling is set. Garnish with pecan halves,
spaced evenly and clock-like around each pie.

Yield: 2 pies. Trust me, you'll be needing them!

NUTRI-NOTE:
One half-cup of
pumpkin daily
may lower the
risk of lung
cancer by half.

*"Let nothing that can be treated by diet
be treated by any other means."*

Dr. Moses Maimonides

Raisin Nut Balls

1 C Brazil nuts, chopped
1 C pecans
1 C walnuts
2 C raisins
2 T honey
1/2 C raw hulled sesame seeds

Soak raisins in water to cover for 1-2 hours.
Place all ingredients except sesame seeds into
processor and chop coarsely.   Mixture will be
thick. Form into 1 inch balls. Roll in sesame
seeds.

Yield: Approximately 36 pieces

*"Eating right means eating naturally. It means
that all foods and drinks consumed should
be as close to their natural state as possible."*

Dr. Cass Ingram

Raspberry Torte

Crust:

2 C raw walnuts
8 pitted dates
1/4 tsp vanilla
2 tsp water

In a food processor use the S blade to process the walnuts until uniformly fine. Add dates, vanilla and water and process until the mixture is sticky. Press into 9 by 7 by 1 inch brownie pan.

Topping:

1 C fresh raspberries
3/4 C unsweetened raspberry preserves
3 T flaxseeds, finely ground

Mix flaxseeds and preserves. Spread in layer over the crust. Top with raspberries.

Yield: 1 torte (approximately 8 servings)

"A diet high in fruits and vegetables is associated with a lower risk of 15 types of cancer, among them colon, breast, cervix and lung."

Andrew Weil, MD

Raw Berry Shortcake

Crust:

2 C almonds
1/3 C honey

Process almonds until finely chopped. Add honey. Knead until well blended. Add a few drops of water if needed to moisten crust, and press into bottom of a 6 by 9 by 2 inch pan.

Topping:

1 C walnuts
1/4 C honey
3 T unsweetened grated coconut
3 dozen strawberries

Cut one dozen strawberries into thin slices and place over crust in a single flat layer. Blend walnuts and coconut until smooth. Spread over strawberry layer. Halve the remaining strawberries, and place, rounded side up, over the entire surface of the cake. Chill for at least 30 minutes before serving.

Yield: Approximately 1 dozen servings

"If a food will not rot or sprout, throw it out."

Patrick Quillin, PhD

Rice Pudding

1 1/2 C cooked short or medium grain brown rice
1/3 C almond milk
1/4 C maple syrup
1/4 tsp cinnamon
2 tsp vanilla extract
1/8 tsp sea salt
1/4 C raisins

Place rice in a large saucepan. Pour in almond milk and stir. Bring mixture up to a boil, then down to a simmer. Add raisins, vanilla, salt and maple syrup. Simmer, stirring often, until liquid thickens to a pudding-like consistency (about 10 minutes). Add cinnamon and stir. Allow to cool. Place in dessert bowls and refrigerate.

Yield: 2 servings

TASTY TIP:
Vanilla rice milk may be substituted for the almond milk, and honey may be substituted for the maple syrup.

"While it is true that cooked and processed foods SUSTAIN life, nevertheless that does not mean that they have the power to regenerate the atoms which furnish the life force to our body."

Norman Walker, DSc, PhD

Stuffed Dates

18 Deglet Noor dates, pitted
1 C almond butter
1/2 C shredded unsweetened coconut
18 pecan halves (optional)

Fill dates generously with nut butter. Roll top of date in coconut. Press a pecan half into top of each date, if desired.

Yield: 18 pieces

"The more a man follows Nature, and is obedient to her laws, the longer he will live; the further he deviates from these the shorter will be his existence."

Christolph Von Hufeland, MD

Vanilla Fudge Ice Cream

2 T raw carob powder, sifted
1 T warm water
4 large ripe bananas, frozen
1/4 tsp vanilla extract
1 tsp honey
1/4 C pecans, chopped
2 T flaxseeds, finely ground
2 strawberries

Mix carob powder with warm water until smooth.
Stir in vanilla and honey. Process frozen
bananas through Champion Juicer using the solid
plate. Gently swirl in the carob mixture. Spoon
into small dessert bowls. Sprinkle with pecans
and flaxseeds. Garnish with strawberry and
serve immediately.

Yield: 2 servings

"Nature cures when given the opportunity."

Dr. Bernard Jensen

JUICES & SMOOTHIES

Almond Coconut Shake

2/3 C raw almonds
1/3 C unsweetened coconut, shredded
1 ripe banana
1 T honey
1/2 tsp vanilla extract
1/4 tsp almond extract
1 1/2 C water

Soak almonds overnight in water to cover. Drain.
Combine water, honey, vanilla and almond extract
in a blender. Slowly add almonds, coconut, and
banana to mixture and blend thoroughly until
smooth.

Yield: 2 cups

NUTRI-NOTE:
This is an
excellent, filling,
morning protein
drink.

*"The present essentially enzyme-less diet is the
parent...of a multitude of our health problems."*

Dr. Edward Howell

Apple-Strawberry Drink

6 apples, cored and cut into sections
1 C strawberries, stems and leaves removed,
    sliced

Put strawberries through juicer. Juice apples.
Stir gently to combine. Serve chilled.

Yield: 32 oz

NUTRI-NOTE:
Consume
immediately,
or store in
refrigerator and
consume within
12 hours, to
preserve
enzymes intact.

*"In order to regain and maintain the proper
balance of health, most of the food we eat
must contain live, vital, organic elements...
found in fresh, raw vegetables, fruits, nuts
and seeds...."*

Norman Walker, DSc, PhD

Carob Malted

1/4 C flaxseeds
2 1/2 C water
1/2 C pine nuts
2 T unsweetened carob powder
2 T maple syrup
4 dates, pitted
1 tsp vanilla extract

Soak the flaxseeds and dates in 1 C water for 24 hours. Pour into blender and mix thoroughly. Add remaining water and other ingredients to flaxseed mixture and liquify. Chill before serving.

Yield: 2 cups

HELPFUL HINT:
You had better double this recipe — it's delicious!

"If you eat any fruits, vegetables, nuts, seeds, or sprouts on a regular basis, you are receiving all the amino acids necessary for your body to build the protein it needs...."

Harvey Diamond

Carob Milk

1 1/2 C almond milk
3 T unsweetened carob powder
2 T maple syrup

Blend all ingredients together. Serve chilled.

YIELD: 1 1/2 cups

> TASTY TIP:
> To transform this "chocolate" milk into a thicker shake, add 3 ripe bananas and blend until smooth. Yield: 3 cups

"The potential life span should be between 100 and 120 years. If we simply apply what we already know...in the field of nutrition, there is no reason why the present average life span shouldn't almost double."

Dr. Thomas G. Gardner

Carrot Apple Juice

2 apples, cored and sliced into 6 slices each
4 carrots, tops removed, scrubbed and scraped

In a juice extractor, juice apples, then carrots.

Yield: 8 - 10 ounces

*"Most of the food we eat in this country
is of a clogging nature....
We must work with our bodies,
not against them. One perfect way
to do that is to cleanse them, not clog them."*

Harvey Diamond

Carrot-Beet-Cucumber Juice

1 cucumber, peeled and quartered lengthwise
1 small beet, sliced, and tops
1 lb carrots, tops removed

Juice ingredients in order given. Roll beet tops
and push through juicer.

Yield: 16 ounces

NUTRI-NOTE:
There is no better
cleanser for your
liver than fresh
beets.

*"People who live solely on fresh raw foods
supplemented with a sufficient volume and
variety of fresh raw vegetable and fruits juices,
do not develop cancers."*

Norman Walker, DSc, PhD

Carrot Celery Juice

3 stalks celery, with leaves
10 medium carrots, tops removed

Cut celery stalks into quarters. Juice celery, then carrots, and combine.

Yield: 12 ounces

NUTRI-NOTE: Celery is rich in potassium and sodium. Celery juice after a workout is a great electrolyte replacement drink.

"The human body is not designed to digest more than one concentrated food...
at the same time.... Any food that is not a fruit and is not a vegetable is concentrated."

Harvey Diamond

Cleansing Cocktail

8 medium carrots, scrubbed, tops removed
1 C fresh parsley
4 stalks celery

Cut celery stalks into quarters. Juice items in order listed and combine.

Yield: 12 ounces

NUTRI-NOTE:
Raw vegetable cocktails provide a great source of minerals.

" It is dangerous to depend on fragments of food factors as they are synthetically made ...in a laboratory or...mutilated by modern food processing methods. No abundance of one factor, no vitamin, mineral, protein, fat or carbohydrate can make up for the lack of the other factors. All must be present, all must be vital, and the only way... of getting them is from natural foods grown in healthy, complete soils."

Fred Miller, DDS

Coco Loco

1 ripe banana
1/2 C fresh or frozen pineapple
2 oz unsweetened coconut milk
1 T maple syrup
1/2 C crushed ice (optional)

Blend all ingredients except ice until smooth.
Add ice if desired and blend again.

Yield: 10 – 14 ounces

*"The best and most nutritious foods
are not processed in any way."*

John H. Tobe

Cruciferous Surprise

3 kale leaves
1/2 C broccoli florets
1/3 head red cabbage, cut into wedges
2 carrots
2 apples, cut into wedges

Juice the kale first, followed by the broccoli and cabbage. Then juice the carrots and apples. Stir well.

Yield: 16 ounces

NUTRI-NOTE: This drink is rich in the sulfur-containing compounds of the cruciferous (cabbage) family that help the body detoxify cancer-causing chemicals and hormones.

"All nutritional energy...originates as solar energy that has been captured and stored by green plants."

Andrew Weil, MD

Green Drink

1/4 C fresh parsley
2 apples, cored and cut into wedges
2 kale leaves
1/4 C spinach

Put parsley through juice extractor first; little, if any, juice should come through. Juice one of the apples, kale, and spinach in that order. Juice second apple. Stir and serve immediately.

Yield: 12 ounces

"...Man has overlooked the power of green....
Since the beginning of life on earth, no animal
has been able to live without green"

Yoshihide Hagiwara, MD

Mocha Shake

2 T chopped almonds
2 T raw sunflower seeds
2 T flaxseeds
1 C water
1/2 C fresh apple juice
1 tsp vanilla extract
1/4 tsp nutmeg
1/8 tsp cinnamon
1/2 tsp Sucanat

Process almonds, sunflower seeds and flaxseeds in blender until coarsely ground. With motor running, slowly pour in water through hole in top. Add remaining ingredients and continue blending until frothy. Serve immediately.

Yield: 14 ounces

HELPFUL HINT:
Soaking the nuts and seeds overnight will increase the digestibility of this drink, but be sure to drain off soak liquid and rinse before blending.

"Stomachs shouldn't be garbage cans."

Dr. Robert G. Jackson

Orange Mint Cooler

2 medium oranges
1 lemon
2 tsp dried mint leaves
2 T honey
1 C water

Peel and seed oranges and lemon. Cut into quarters and juice in juice extractor. Pour juice into blender. Add mint and honey and process on high speed until well blended. Add water and process at low speed until smooth. Serve over ice cubes.

Yield: 2 cups

TASTY TIP:
Fresh mint leaves make an attractive garnish, and 4 teaspoons may be substituted for the dried leaves.

"Food is a love note from God....It says I love you and I shall take care of you and sustain you with the offerings of My earth."

Gabriel Cousens, MD

Papaya Maya

1 ripe banana
1/2 C fresh or frozen papaya chunks
1 C apple juice
1 tsp maple syrup

Blend all ingredients until smooth. Serve chilled.

Yield: 14 ounces

TASTY TIP:
For variation, use almond milk in place of apple juice.

"Progressive degeneration of the cells and tissues follows the continuous consumption of cooked and processed foods."

Norman Walker, DSc, PhD

Peaches and Cream

1 ripe banana
1 C fresh peaches, peeled, or frozen peaches
1/4 C vanilla yogurt (preferably goat's milk)
1/2 C apple juice, rice milk or goat's milk
1 1/2T maple syrup
1/2 C ice (optional)

Blend all ingredients except ice until smooth.
Add ice if desired and blend again.

Yield: approximately 16 ounces

TASTY TIP:
The amount of maple syrup should be adjusted, depending on whether the liquid is apple juice or milk.

*"Eating close to nature
is definitely a key to wellness."*

Sherry Rogers, MD

Pink Lemonade

2 fresh lemons, peeled and quartered
1/2 C fresh dark cherries, pitted
1/4 C honey
1 C water

Juice lemons and cherries. Pour mixture into blender. Add honey and water and blend well. Pour over ice cubes and serve.

Yield: 14 ounces

"Juicing is a phenomenal way to reach the goal of ingesting 60% of total calories from raw foods."

Michael Murray, ND

Sesame Shake

1 C almond milk
3 T hulled sesame seeds
1 ripe banana
1/2 tsp vanilla extract

Pour sesame seeds into coffee mill and grind to a
fine powder. Transfer to blender along with
banana, vanilla, and 1/4 C almond milk. Blend on
high, slowly adding remaining milk, until smooth.
Chill.

Yield: 12 ounces

NUTRI-NOTE:
Sesame seeds
are excellent for
strength and
rebuilding.

*"If people would only learn to eat properly,
they could live the best years of their lives
twice over."*

Richard M. Field, MD

Strawberry Milk

1/2 C vanilla flavored goat milk yogurt
4 oz apple juice
1/2 C strawberries, sliced
1 tsp maple syrup
1/4 tsp vanilla extract

Blend all ingredients together until smooth.

Yield: approximately 12 ounces

NUTRI-NOTE:
Goat's milk is more digestible than cow's milk because it is similar to human breast milk.

"The cooking, heating, processing, fragmenting and refining of foods not only destroys much of their nutritional value, but also turns some of them into actually toxic substances."

John H. Tobe

Sunflower Seed Milk

1 C raw sunflower seeds
2 1/4 C cold water
1 T maple syrup
1 T vanilla
10 Deglet Noor dates, pitted and chopped
dash cinnamon

Place seeds, maple syrup, vanilla and 1 C water in
blender and blend until smooth. Add dates and
blend for 1 minute. Slowly add remaining water
and blend again.

Yield: 2 3/4 cups

NUTRI-NOTE:
Raw sunflower
seeds are an
excellent source
of zinc,
supportive of
wound healing
and prostate
health.

*"The miracle of the age is that we are as
well as we are with the mutilation going on
with the foods that we eat."*

Dr. Bernard Jensen

Tango Mango

1 ripe banana
1 C frozen mango cubes
6 oz apple juice or orange juice
1 T maple syrup
1/2 C ice (optional)

Blend all ingredients except ice together until smooth. If desired, add ice and reblend.

Yield: 14 – 16 ounces

"People who eat [a plant-based diet] over long periods of time or even lifetimes have no protein problems. The Hunzas,...Asians, and half a billion Hindus eat very little protein food...yet have no protein deficiencies."

Harvey Diamond

Tropical Smoothie

1/4 ripe medium avocado
1/2 C ripe papaya chunks
1/2 C fresh coconut juice
1 ripe banana
1 T honey

Blend all ingredients together until creamy smooth.

Yield: 12 ounces

HELPFUL HINT:
If fresh coconut juice is unavailable, use a non-sulfite canned coconut milk like Thai Kitchen Lite, plus 2 T water.

"The basic key to the efficacy of nourishing your body is the LIFE which is present in your food...."

Norman Walker, DSc, PhD

Velvety Cashew Milk

1/3 C raw cashews
3/4 C water
2 T maple syrup
1/2 tsp vanilla extract

Grind cashews in coffee grinder to achieve a fine powder. Place in blender with water, maple syrup and vanilla. Process on medium to a smooth consistency.

Yield: 8 ounces

HELPFUL HINT:
Larger quantities may be stored in refrigerator for 4 days.

"No food was ever nutritionally improved by cooking."

John H. Tobe

Very Berry

1 ripe banana
1/2 C frozen or fresh strawberries, chopped
1/2 C frozen or fresh raspberries
1 C apple juice, rice milk or almond milk
2 T maple syrup
1/2 C crushed ice (optional)

Blend all ingredients except ice until smooth.
Add ice if desired and blend again.

Yield: approximately 16 ounces

TASTY TIP:
For variety,
substitute rice
milk or almond
milk for apple
juice, and use
2T maple syrup.

*"The fact that for generations, millions upon
millions of people have lived...who have rarely
if ever eaten anything but cooked foods
does not prove that their being alive
is the result of eating cooked foods."*

Norman Walker, DSc, PhD

Walnut Date Milk

1 qt water
1/4 C honey
1 C walnuts, finely ground
1 C dates, pitted

Pour 1 C water into blender. Add other ingredients and blend at medium speed. With blender running, gradually add remaining water and increase speed until liquified.

Yield: 5 cups

NUTRI-NOTE:
Raw walnuts are a good source of immune-boosting omega-3 fatty acids.

"Nature struggles...to keep us well at all times, and failure to accomplish this end is due mainly to the fact that we have thrown in her way too many impediments in the form of wrong foods, deficient foods, imbalanced foods, refined foods, too much food...."

William Howard Hay, MD

Watermelon Cooler

1 lemon, peeled
7 C small chunks ripe watermelon

Slowly feed watermelon chunks into juicer. Juice lemon. Stir together well. Serve chilled.

Yield: About 3 1/2 cups

NUTRI-NOTE:
This drink is a great kidney detoxifier, as watermelon is an excellent diuretic.

"Let your food be your medicine and your medicine your food."

Hippocrates

POSTSCRIPT

It is my sincere hope that this book will help you make a lifetime commitment to healthful eating.

As you change over to a plant-based diet consisting primarily of uncooked whole foods, don't concentrate on what you have to give up; that's negative and disempowering thinking. Rather, **focus on what to include**. Basically, if you aim to consume 10 servings (think half-cup to fist-size) of fresh fruits and vegetables daily, you won't have a lot of room – or time – to eat too much of the poor quality foods. In fact, you probably won't even desire them.

One of the best ways of optimizing your intake of fruits and veggies is juicing, of course. But if the juicing and the 10 servings sound a bit daunting, you should at least consider taking Juice Plus+, which represents the dehydrated juices of 17 different fruits and vegetables in capsule form. It certainly is not a substitute for proper eating, but a great supplement to help with the transition.

Do remember to be kind to yourself. Give yourself permission not to be perfect, for **health is not about perfection; it is about balance**. Guilt is a useless emotion anyway, and the only thing more dangerous to your health than what you're eating is what's eating you. If you're going to eat something "bad," please enjoy the heck out of it – and then get back to your health program.

Think of nutritional improvement as rungs on a very tall ladder. The climb should be a gradual process, and once you leave the ground, you should be proud of each additional step you take. Do not allow yourself to become overwhelmed, or you might give up. After all, *you* want to be in control of your self-help program; you don't want *it* to control *you.* Know that you cannot make all of the changes at once, and perhaps some you will never make. So **choose your battles**, and do not attempt to fight the next one until you have mastered the previous one – whether it takes a few days, a few weeks or a few months.

Be aware that as you ease the toxic food habits out of your life, their residues will need to be eased out of your body. When you make significant changes in your dietary habits, your body may thank you in some uncomfortable ways: fatigue, runny nose, rash, headache, diarrhea, swollen glands, flu-like symptoms, even fever. This "healing crisis," as it is sometimes called, may happen in a few weeks or months or not at all. It should be short-lived, though, and followed by a period of feeling better than you have in quite some time.

The recipes in this book represent the foods I have been eating almost exclusively for over a quarter of a century. Despite the fact that I still have more rungs to climb, I have three times the energy now that I had when I was one-third my age! Yes, I do cheat occasionally, but I notice that the foods I love don't always love me back. So when friends admire my dietary discipline, I explain that it's not so much discipline as it is just dislike for how I feel when I cheat.

That is my wish for you – a feeling of such vibrant health that once you experience it, you won't want to be without it!

REFERENCES

Albright, Nancy, *The Rodale Cookbook*, Rodale, Emmaus, PA, 1973

Barefoot, Robert, *Death by Diet*, Triad, Southeastern, PA, 2002

Barnard, Neal, *Food For Life*, Crown, NY, 1993

_____ *The Power of Your Plate*, Book Publishing, Summertown, TN, 1995

Biehler, Henry, *Food is Your Best Medicine*, Random House, NY, 1965

Boutenko, Sergei and Valya, *Eating Without Heating*, Raw Family, Ashland, OR, 2002

Calabro, Rose Lee, *Living in the Raw*, Rose, Santa Cruz, 1998

Carper, Jean, *The Food Pharmacy*, Bantam, New York, 1988

Cousens, Gabriel, *Conscious Eating*, North Atlantic, Berkeley, CA, 2000

Diamond, Harvey and Marilyn, *Fit for Life*, Warner, NY, 1985

Eaton , S. Boyd and Konner, Melvin, "Paleolithic Nutrition, *New England Journal of Medicine* 313:283-89, 1985

Eaton, S. Boyd, Shostak, Marjorie, and Konner, Melvin, *Paleolithic Prescription*, Harper & Row, New York, 1988

Emeka, Mauris, *Cancer's Best Medicine*, Apollo, Port Orchard, WA, 2004

Fallon, Sally, *Nourishing Traditions*, ProMotion, San Diego, 1995

Grossman, Ruth and Bob, *The Italian-Kosher Cookbook*, Paul S. Eriksson, New York, 1964

Heber, David,*What Color is Your Diet?* HarperCollins, New York, 2001

Howell, Edward, *Enzyme Nutrition*, Avery, Wayne, NJ, 1985

Hunsberger, Eydie Mae, *Eydie Mae's Natural Recipes*, Avery, Wayne, NJ, 1978

Ingram, Cass, *Eat Right or Die Young*, Literary Visions, Cedar Rapids, IA, 1989

Jack, Alex, ed., *Let Food Be Thy Medicine*, One Peaceful World, Becket, MA, 1991

Jensen, Bernard, *Vital Foods for Total Health*, Solana Beach, CA, 1984

Malkmus, George, *God's Way to Ultimate Health*, Hallelujah Acres, Eidson, TN, 1995

Mercola, Joseph, *Dr. Mercola's Total Health Cookbook & Program*, Mercola.com, Schaumberg, IL, 2003

_____ *The No-Grain Diet*, Dutton/Penguin Group, New York, 2003

Murray, Michael,*The Complete Book of Juicing*, Prima, Roseville, CA, 1992

Null, Gary, *The Joy of Juicing*, Avery, New York, 1992

Peary, M. Warren, *The 10 Biggest Diet Myths That Ruin Your Health*, American Institute for Abundant Living, Santa Fe, NM, 2003

Pirello, Christina, *Glow*, Berkeley, New York, 2001

Pitchford, Paul, *Healing With Whole Foods*, North Atlantic, Berkeley, CA, 1993

Quillin, Patrick, *Beating Cancer With Nutrition*, Nutrition Times, Tulsa, OK, 2001

Rhio, *Hooked on Raw*, Beso, NY, 2000

Rogers, Sherry, *You Are What You Ate*, Prestige, Syracuse, NY, 2000

Romano, Rita, *Dining in the Raw*, Kensington , New York, 1992

Shannon, Nomi, *The Raw Gourmet*, Alive, Nurnaby, BC, 1999

Sokosh, Doris, *My Recipes for Recovery*, FACT, New Canaan, CT, 1990

Sparandeo, James, *Scientific Relationships Between Diet and Cancer Survival*, Comprehensive Nutritional News, West Long Branch, NJ, 1991

Spitler, Sue, 1001 Low-Fat Vegetarian Recipes, Surry, Chicago, 1997

Tobe, John H., *No-Cook Book*, The Provoker, St. Catharines, Ontario, Canada, 1969

Waerland, Ebba, *Rebuilding Health*, Arco, New York, 1972

Walker, Norman, *Fresh Vegetable and Fruit Juices*, Norwalk, Prescott, AZ, 1978

Wasserman, Debra, *The Low Fat Jewish Vegetarian Cookbook*, The Vegetarian Resource Group, Baltimore, 1994

Weil, Andrew, *Eating Well for Optimum Health*, HarperCollins, New York, 2001

Wigmore, Ann, *The Hippocrates Diet and Health Program*, Avery, Wayne, NJ, 1984

RECIPE INDEX